SILENT MYOCARDIAL ISCHEMIA

DEVELOPMENTS IN CARDIOVASCULAR MEDICINE

Morganroth, Joel, Moore, E.N., eds.: Sudden cardiac death and congestive heart failure: Diagnosis and treatment. 1983. ISBN 0-89838-580-6.
Perry, H.M., ed.: Lifelong management of hypertension. ISBN 0-89838-582-2.
Jaffe, E.A., ed.: Biology of endothelial cells. ISBN 0-89838-587-3.
Surawicz, B., Reddy, C.P., Prystowsky, E.N., eds.: Tachycardias. 1984. ISBN 0-89838-588-1.
Spencer, M.P., ed.: Cardiac Doppler diagnosis. ISBN 0-89838-591-1.
Villareal, H.V., Sambhi, M.P., eds.: Topics in pathophysiology of hypertension. ISBN 0-89838-595-4.
Messerli, F.H., ed.: Cardiovascular disease in the elderly. 1984. ISBN 0-89838-596-2.
Simoons, M.L., Reiber, J.H.C., eds.: Nuclear imaging in clinical cardiology. ISBN 0-89838-599-7.
Ter Keurs, H.E.D.J., Schipperheym, J.J., eds.: Cardiac left ventricular hypertrophy. ISBN 0-89838-612-8.
Sperelakis, N., ed.: Physiology and pathophysiology of the heart. ISBN 0-89838-615-2.
Messerli, F.H., ed.: Kidney in essential hypertension. 1983. ISBN 0-89838-616-0.
Sambhi, M.P., ed.: Fundamental fault in hypertension. ISBN 0-89838-638-1.
Marchesi, D., ed.: Ambulatory monitoring: Cardiovascular system and allied applications. ISBN 0-89838-642-X.
Kupper, W., Macalpin, R.N., Bleifeld, W., eds.: Coronary tone in ischemic heart disease. ISBN 0-89838-646-2.
Sperelakis, N., Caulfield, J.B., eds.: Calcium antagonists: Mechanisms of action on cardiac muscle and vascular smooth muscle. ISBN 0-89838-655-1.
Godfraind, T., Herman, A.S., Wellens, D., eds.: Entry blockers in cardiovascular and cerebral dysfunctions. ISBN 0-89838-658-6.
Morganroth, J., Moore, E.N., eds.: Interventions in the acute phase of myocardial infarction. ISBN 0-89838-659-4.
Abel, F.L., Newman, W.H., eds.: Functional aspects of the normal, hypertrophied, and failing heart. ISBN 0-89838-665-9.
Sideman, S., and Beyar, R., eds.: Simulation and imaging of the cardiac system. ISBN 0-89838-687-X.
van de Wall, E., Lie, K.I., eds.: Recent views on hypertrophic cardiomyopathy. ISBN 0-89838-694-2.
Beamish, R.E., Singal, P.K., Dhalla, N.S., eds.: Stress and heart disease. ISBN 089838-709-4.
Beamish, R.E., Panagia, V., Dhalla, N.S., eds.: Pathogenesis of stress-induced heart disease. ISBN 0-89838-710-8.
Morganroth, J., Moore, E.N., eds., Cardiac arrhythmias: New therapeutic drugs and devices. ISBN 0-89838-716-7.
Mathes, P., ed.: Secondary prevention in coronary artery disease and myocardial infarction. ISBN 0-89838-736-1.
Stone, H. Lowell, Weglicki, W.B., eds.: Pathology of cardiovascular injury. ISBN 0-89838-743-4.
Meyer, J., Erbel, R., Rupprecht, H.J., eds.: Improvement of myocardial perfusion. ISBN 0-89838-748-5.
Reiber, J.H.C., Serruys, P.W., Slager, C.J.: Quantitative coronary and left ventricular cineangiography. ISBN 0-89838-760-4.
Fagard, R.H., Bekaert, I.E., eds.: Sports Cardiology. ISBN 0-89838-782-5.
Reiber, J.H.C., Serruys, P.W., eds.: State of the art in quantitative coronary arteriography. ISBN 0-89838-804-X.
Roelandt, J., ed.: Color doppler flow imaging. ISBN 0-89838-806-6.
van de Wall, E.E., ed.: Noninvasive imaging of cardiac metabolism. ISBN 0-89838-812-0.
Liebman, J., Plonsey, R., Rudy, Y., eds.: Pediatric and fundamental electrocardiography. ISBN 0-89838-815-5.
Higler, H., Hombach, V., eds.: Invasive cardiovascular therapy. ISBN 0-89838-818-X.
Serruys, P.W., Meester, G.T., eds.: Coronary angioplasty: a controlled model for ischemia. ISBN 0-89838-819-8.
Tooke, J.E., Smaje, L.H., eds.: Clinical investigation of the microcirculation. ISBN 0-89838-833-3.
van Dam, Th., van Oosterom, A., eds.: Electrocardiographic body surface mapping. ISBN 0-89838-834-1.
Spencer, M.P., ed.: Ultrasonic diagnosis of cerebrovascular disease. ISBN 0-89838-836-8.
Legato, M.J., ed.: The stressed heart. ISBN 0-89838-848-X.
Safar, M.E., ed.: Arterial and venous systems in essential hypertension. ISBN 0-89838-857-0.
Roelandt, J., ed.: Digital techniques in echocardiography. ISBN 0-89838-861-9.
Morganroth, J., Moore, E.N., eds.: Silent myocardial ischemia. ISBN 0–89838–380–3.

SILENT MYOCARDIAL ISCHEMIA

Proceedings of the Symposium on New Drugs and Devices
October 15–16, 1987, Philadelphia, Pennsylvania

edited by:

Joel Morganroth, M.D.
Likoff Cardiovascular Institute
Hahnemann Medical College and Hospital

and

E. Neil Moore
School of Veterinary Medicine
University of Pennsylvania

Kluwer Academic Publishers
Boston/Dordrecht/Lancaster

Distributors for North America:
Kluwer Academic Publishers
101 Philip Drive
Assinippi Park
Norwell, Massachusetts 02061, USA

Distributors for the UK and Ireland:
Kluwer Academic Publishers
Falcon House, Queen Square
Lancaster LA1 1RN, UNITED KINGDOM

Distributors for all other countries:
Kluwer Academic Publishers Group
Distribution Centre
Post Office Box 322
3300 AH Dordrecht, THE NETHERLANDS

Library of Congress Cataloging-in-Publication Data

Symposium on New Drugs and Devices (8th : 1987 :
Philadelphia, Pa.)
Silent myocardial ischemia.

(Developments in cardiovascular medicine ; 88)
1. Coronary heart disease—Congresses. 2. Ischemia—
Congresses. I. Morganroth, Joel. II. Moore, E. Neil.
III. Title. IV. Series: Development in cardiovascular
medicine ; v. 88. [DNLM: 1. Coronary Disease—drug
therapy—congresses. 2. Coronary Disease—physiopathology—
congresses. 3. Longitudinal Studies—congresses.
W1 DE997VME v. 88 / WG 300 S98925 1987s]
RC685.C6S94 1987 616.1'23 88-8922
ISBN 0-89838-380-3

Printed in the United States of America

CONTENTS

III TRIAL DESIGNS

IV THERAPY AND FDA CLAIMS

V COMBINATION DRUG THERAPY—FDA ISSUES

SYMPOSIUM ON NEW DRUGS AND DEVICES

OCTOBER 15 - 16, 1987

FACULTY

J. Thomas Bigger, Jr., M.D.
Department of Medicine
Columbia University Health Sciences
630 West 168th Street
New York, NY 10032
(212) 305-4093

Peter F. Cohn, M.D.
Professor of Medicine
Chief, Cardiology Division
S.U.N.Y. Health Sciences Center at Stony Brook
Room T-17-020
SUNY Health Sciences Center
Stony Brook, NY 11794
(516) 444-1060

William Frishman, M.D.
Professor of Medicine
Albert Einstein College of Medicine
1825 Eastchester Road
Bronx, NY 10461
(212) 904-2896

Robert S. Gibson, M.D.
Associate Professor of Medicine
Director, Cardiac Noninvasive Laboratory
University of Virginia
Box 468
Medical Center, University of Virginia
Charlottesville, VA 22908
(804) 924-2930

Sidney O. Gottlieb, M.D.
Assistant Professor of Medicine
Johns Hopkins University School of Medicine
Division of Cardiology
B-1 South
Francis Scott Key Medical Center
4940 Eastern Avenue
Baltimore, MD 21224
(301) 955-0856

Leonard N. Horowitz, M.D.
Director, Cardiac Electrophysiology
and Electrocardiography
Presbyterian-University of Penn. Med. Ctr.
39th & Market Streets
Philadelphia, PA 19104
(215) 662-9097

Harold L. Kennedy, M.D., MPH
Professor
Chief, Division of Cardiology
St. Louis University School of Medicine
1325 S. Grand Blvd.
St. Louis, MO 63104
(314) 577-8890

Raymond J. Lipicky, M.D.
Director of the Division of
Cardio-Renal Drug Products
Food and Drug Administration
HFN-110, Room 16B45
5600 Fishers Lane
Rockville, MD 20857
(301) 443-4730

Joel Morganroth, M.D.
Prof. of Med. & Pharm., Hahnemann Univ.
Dir., Cardiac Res. & Develop., The Graduate Hosp.
The Graduate Hospital
One Graduate Plaza
Philadelphia, PA 19146
(215) 893-2000

E. Neil Moore, DVM, Ph.D.
Professor of Physiology in Medicine
University of Pennsylvania
School of Veterinary Medicine
3800 Spruce Street
Philadelphia, PA 19104
(215) 898-8897

Carl J. Pepine
Professor of Medicine
J277 University of Florida
Gainesville, FL 32610
(904) 374-6052

Bertram Pitt, M.D.
Professor of Internal Medicine
Director, Cardiology Division
University of Michigan Med. Ctr.
1500 E. Medical Center Drive
3910 Taubman
Ann Arbor, MI 48109-0366
(313) 936-5255

Dr. Stephen Scheidt
Professor of Clinical Medicine
The New York Hospital-Cornell Med. Ctr.
525 East 68th Street
New York, NY 10021
(212) 472-4900

Andrew P. Selwyn, M.D.
Physician, Director of Cardiac Cath.
Division of Cardiology
Brigham & Women's Hospital
75 Francis Street
Boston, MA 02115
(617) 732-7136

Robert Temple, M.D.
Director, Office of Drug Research & Review
Food and Drug Administration
5600 Fishers Lane
Rockville, MD 20857
(301) 443-4330

Donald A. Weiner, M.D.
Associate Professor of Medicine
Boston University Medical School
University Hospital
75 East Newton Street
Boston, MA 02118
(617) 638-8700

PREFACE

Although some investigators have questioned the importance and even the existence of silent myocardial ischemia, documentation presented at this two day symposium leaves little doubt about its existence and importance. It has been estimated that about 3 million of the estimated 4 million angina sufferers in the United States have frequent episodes of silent myocardial ischemia. Although it is not possible to define how many Americans die due to silent ischemia, it has been suggested that the mortality rate may exceed hundreds of thousands of victims annually. Unfortunately, there still remains a lack of definitive information as to why some ischemic events are painless. Some suggest the concept that the location and size of the myocardium at jeopardy relates to pain, that the pain threshold varies from patient to patient or that there are neurological deficits in the myocardium of some patients with silent ischemia. Abnormalities in myocardial perfusion and function can occur without pain. An interesting observation presented by several investigators has been that when a coronary artery is occluded in man, no ischemic pain is perceived for the first 30 seconds. Only after a 30 second period or so of occlusion does angina occur. An even more confusing observation is that some 30 second periods of occlusion of the same vessel in the same patient results in angina while the next occlusion can be a totally silent event.

Clearly, brief ischemic events may not result in pain, but why prolon ged ischemic events have variable perception of pain is a question that needs to be answered.

A number of techniques are capable of identifying silent myocardial ischemia including Holter monitoring, exercise testing and radionuclide techniques. False positives do occur with each test and there is no solid gold standard for identifying silent ischemia since even the radionuclide thallium perfusion can provide erroneous diagnoses of silent myocardial ischemia.

One of the most important questions regarding silent myocardial ischemia is "how aggressive should the treatment for silent myocardial ischemia be, if any"? We are not definitely certain that decreasing the incidence of silent myocardial ischemia, or for that matter decreasing the incidence of angina per se, will necessarily decrease mortality. It is conceivable that silent ischemic events can result in enhanced coronary collateralization which in turn might improve the likelihood of a patient surviving a given ischemic event.

While currently available anti-angina agents are usually effective for decreasing angina events, the indications and guidelines for a claim for treatment of silent ischemia from the Food and Drug Administration are not clear. Clinical research studies should aim to demonstrate that an anti-anginal drug is also anti-ischemic and a silent ischemia claim will undoubtedly have to show that reducing such events will impact at least on patient morbidity if not mortality.

Silent myocardial ischemia is an important medical problem. However its detection and medical impact remain to be fully elucidated. Perhaps it is artificial to categorize ischemia into silent and symptomatic forms since ischemia, whatever its presentation, impairs myocardial integrity.

This symposium has brought together Food and Drug Administration regulators, pharmaceutical and academic scientists who all debated the current state-of-the-art and future directions of this critical problem. The following pages represent these issues and it is hoped that this information will guide the reader to a clearer understanding of the status and direction of this medical problem.

I. EPIDEMIOLOGY, PATHOPHYSIOLOGY, CLASSIFICATION

1

EPIDEMIOLOGY AND PREVALENCE OF SILENT MYOCARDIAL ISCHEMIA, AND PROGNOSIS IN ASYMPTOMATIC PATIENTS

PETER F. COHN

Cardiology Division, Department of Medicine, State University of New York Health Sciences Center, Stony Brook, New York

Although heart disease is the nation's number one killer, its presentation can take many forms. Some of these have only recently received the attention they deserve. For example, textbooks traditionally teach us that the natural history of coronary artery disease proceeds in an orderly fashion from a presymptomatic phase to angina to myocardial infarction to death. This is a stereotypical presentation that is not borne out by the facts. Data from epidemiologic surveys - such as the Framingham Study - suggest that for every individual who presents with angina, there is another one whose first manifestation of disease is either a myocardial infarction or sudden death. Autopsy studies performed in several centers over the last decade indicate that many of those who have sudden death as their first manifestation of coronary artery disease have had episodes of unrecognized infarction prior to the fatal event. Similarly, there is also data showing that prior painless ischemic events occur in patients who present with infarctions without antecedent angina.

Silent (painless) myocardial ischemia is defined as objective evidence of myocardial ischemia (via direct or indirect measurements of left ventricular function, perfusion, metabolism or electrical activity) without chest pain or other anginal equivalents. It can occur in a variety of settings and the numbers of patients can be quite large. We have estimated there are 1-2 million middle-aged men in the United States with totally asymptomatic coronary artery disease (defined as Type 1 in our classification system), 50,000 new cases of post-infarction silent ischemia per year (Type 2) and at least 2 million patients with both angina and silent ischemia (Type 3). Estimating the prevalence of silent myocardial ischemia requires accurate methods of detection. At present, the detection of silent ischemia depends largely on the use of ambulatory ECG monitoring, exercise ECGs, as well as related exercise radionuclide or echocardiographic procedures. The clinical features of patients with silent myocardial ischemia are very similar to those with symptomatic coronary artery disease, including conventional risk factors, number of vessels diseased, abnormalities of left ventricular function, stress test results, etc.

Several studies have addressed prognosis in the different types of patients with silent myocardial ischemia. Prognostic studies in asymptomatic persons are either epidemiologic or anatomic. Only the latter have arteriographic data, though both employ exercise tests. Anatomic studies provide arteriographic evidence that the ECG and perfusion abnormalities are associated with discrete coronary stenoses. Recent surveys of the epidemiologic type are the MRFIT Study and the Lipid Research Clinics Mortality Follow-Up Study. In the latter, for example, a positive exercise test was associated with a cumulative mortality of 11.9% over 8.1 years mean follow-up time, versus 1.2% over 8.6 years for men with a negative test. The best of the angiographic studies is the one from Norway. Fifty patients have been followed for over 12 years. Mortality in the three vessel disease subgroup was 3% per year with an even higher morbidity rate. Thus, of the 17 men with three-vessel disease, six had died (two suddenly), four of the survivors had non-fatal myocardial infarctions, seven others developed angina and 10 had worsening of the ECG responses on their stress test. Progression of the angiographic lesions on repeat coronary angiography was another common finding in survivors.

Sudden death has also been associated with Type 1 silent ischemia. About 50,000 of the 250,000 sudden death victims in this country per year have no prior history of heart disease, yet as noted earlier, when autopsies are performed, these apparently healthy persons have evidence of advanced arteriosclerotic disease in their coronary arteries, and scars in their myocardium.

This brief summary has highlighted the magnitude of the problem and indicated some of its prognostic implications. In my opinion, continued, intensive research in this area is essential for a fuller understanding of this important medical and public health problem.

References

1. Cohn PF. Silent Myocardial Ischemia and Infarction, New York: Marcel Dekker, 1986.

2

PATHOPHYSIOLOGY OF ISCHEMIA : WHY ARE SOME EPISODES SILENT ?

CARL PEPINE, MD
Division of Cardiology, Department of Medicine, University of Florida, Gainesville, Florida

ABSTRACT

Myocardial ischemia occurring during daily life is characterized by a high frequency of silent ischemic episodes. Asymptomatic patients with severe coronary artery disease have only silent episodes while most symptomatic patients have both painful and silent episodes, with silent being prevalent. The extent and severity of coronary artery disease in asymptomatic patients is similar to that found in the symptomatic patients. In the symptomatic patients the silent episodes are accompanied by objective markers of ischemia that indicate that the silent episodes are as severe as the painful episodes. The silent episodes have a characteristic circadian variation with highest frequency between 6 AM and noon and lowest frequency between midnight and 6 AM. Silent episodes also occur at heart rate and activity levels lower than those achieved during exercise-induced angina, suggesting that myocardial oxygen supply is temporarily reduced. Recent data also suggests sympathetic activation and rise in heart rate occur during silent ischemic episodes. This would increase myocardial oxygen demand. All of these findings indicate that both supply- and demand-side mechanisms are important in the pathophysiology of silent ischemia.

INTRODUCTION

Objective evidence for transient myocardial ischemia

occurs very frequently in the absence of symptoms. This syndrome, termed silent or painless myocardial ischemia as opposed to painful ischemia (eg, angina or its equivalents), occurs in patients with all of the usual symptomatic forms of coronary artery disease (eg, angina, myocardial infarction and sudden death) as well as in those who may be in a totally asymptomatic phase. This report will review the pathophysiologic aspects of silent and painful ischemia.

PATHOPHYSIOLOGY

The basic process through which coronary artery disease produces morbidity and mortality and alters quality of life is myocardial ischemia. Traditionally, it has been accepted that ischemia results when the myocardial oxygen supply-demand relationship decreases to a critical level in a region of the left ventricle. Myocardial oxygen supply is determined largely by oxygen delivered via coronary blood flow. Myocardial oxygen delivery is controlled by factors that regulate coronary flow; factors determined by hydraulic and anatomic factors. The hydraulic factors include: coronary perfusion pressure, which is related to systemic blood pressure, the left ventricular diastolic pressure, and the time available for diastolic coronary flow (eg, diastolic filling period which is inversely proportional to heart rate). The anatomic factors are determined by the caliber of the arteriolar bed and the large coronary arteries. Coronary vessel size is controlled by a number of factors that influence vascular smooth muscle activation. Vasoconstrictors (eg, norepinephrine, ATP) may act through medial receptors or through recently demonstrated endothelial mechanisms. Acetylcholine and 5-HT release one or several endothelial derived factors (EDRF) which relax coronary vascular smooth muscle to dilate coronary arteries. One of these factors appears to be nitrous oxide which in turn mediates smooth muscle relaxation through endogenous cGMP generation to act in a manner analogous to exogenously administered organic nitrates. Atherosclerosis (thickened intima and plaque) and probably other processes such as coronary artery spasm and inflammation appear to be associated with various degrees of endothelial dysfunction. Structurally damaged endothelium (eg, plaque rupture and disruption) may enhance platelet aggregation and adherence, fibrin deposition, and nonocclusive thrombus formation. Lack of normal endogenous relaxation-dilatation mechanisms, thrombotic elements, and local release of vasoactive substances (thromboxane, serotonin, leukotrienes, etc) set the stage for reduction of regional blood flow to limit myocardial oxygen delivery in a variable fashion. Some noncoronary factors, such as arterial blood oxygen content and blood viscosity (ie, largely related to fibrinogen concentration), also play an important role. On the other hand, myocardial oxygen demand is mediated by heart rate, contractility, and left ventricular systolic wall stress. The latter is directly related to peak left ventricular pressure (ie, systolic blood pressure in the absence of outflow obstruction) and left ventricular chamber size, and inversely related to left ventricular wall thickness.

The duration and extent of myocardium involved in the supply-demand imbalance are of central importance. Brief periods (several minutes) of temporary decrease in the myocardial oxygen supply-demand ratio promptly result in transient ischemia. Transient ischemia involving a myocardium of a critical size is usually associated with reversible changes of the electrocardiogram (ST segment depression), myocardial blood flow distribution (perfusion deficits), contractile function (dyskinesis), and occasionally a very subjective sensation perceived as chest discomfort (angina pectoris and its equivalents). More prolonged (30 to 60 min) disruptions in the myocardial supply-demand balance, such as that resulting from coronary thrombosis, and perhaps very frequent but briefer episodes, have the potential to result in myocardial injury and necrosis (eg, infarction) or dysrhythmias (eg, ventricular tachycardia) which may lead to death. Under some conditions ischemic injury may produce myocardial dysfunction without necrosis, which persists for a long period after the supply-demand imbalance has been corrected. This phenomenon has been called "myocardial stunning" and has important implications.

Recently ischemia occurring in ambulatory patients has been studied using ST segment depression recorded by ambulatory electrocardiographic monitoring as an objective marker of ischemia. Most ischemia detected during daily life is silent. The precise reason why these episodes are silent is unknown. Certain patients, such as those with diabetes, neuropathy, and cardiac transplantation, appear to be at higher risk for silent ischemia due to cardiac sensory dysfunction. Altered cutaneous sensory function has been suggested in some patients with silent ischemia. An increase in endogenous opiate function has also been reported in some other patients. Nevertheless, silent and painful episodes of ischemia occur at different times in many individuals without known sensory dysfunction. In the latter patients even painful ischemic episodes may be accompanied by relatively long perisymptomatic periods of silent ischemia. Thus, it is unlikely that sensory dysfunction accounts for most episodes of silent ischemia.

Traditional views of the pathophysiology of ischemia have undergone considerable modification in light of recent investigation of ischemia during daily life. Previously, characterization of transient ischemic episodes in the exercise laboratory suggested that the majority of episodes were painful and evoked by increasing myocardial oxygen demands. Since ST segment depression often preceded perception of symptoms in this setting, silent or asymptomatic ischemia was considered a less severe form of ischemia. Considerable data comparing patients with silent and those with painful ischemia, however, shows similar left ventricular dysfunction, severity of coronary artery disease, and other abnormalities. Even when comparing silent with painful episodes in the same individual, there is considerable overlap in the duration and magnitude of ST segment depression as well as other abnormalities related to extent and magnitude of myocardial ischemia. Because the silent ischemic episodes go unrecognized, many episodes are extremely prolonged (> 30 min) and may be associated with signs of more severe ischemia compared with ischemic episodes accompanied by pain.

Individual patients may have ischemic episodes occurring at any time of day, but studies from groups of patients indicate that ischemia appears in a characteristic circadian pattern. Ischemic episodes cluster in a time period beginning shortly after waking (6 AM) and peak at approximately noon. In the period between midnight and 6 AM ischemic episodes are relatively infrequent. This diurnal pattern is similar to that observed for acute myocardial infarction, sudden cardiac death, and thrombotic stroke. This pattern relates temporally to the period of heightened sympathetic activation, and $beta_1$ adrenergic blockade prevents most of this AM increase in ischemia.

The majority of ischemic episodes detected during daily life, in particular the silent episodes, occur at heart rates lower than those reached at the onset of ischemia during exercise testing. This finding, coupled with data indicating that ambulatory blood pressure is not significantly changed before the onset of ischemia during normal life, suggests that myocardial oxygen delivery is reduced at times when most daily ischemic episodes occur. Analysis of patient activities at the onset of ischemia during life reveals relatively low level activities are associated with these episodes. This finding supports the heart rate data suggesting a lower myocardial oxygen demand at the onset of silent episodes compared with painful episodes induced in the exercise laboratory. These results imply that other stressors present in the daily life of these patients, are involved in the provocation of ischemia. Some of these have recently been identified as mental stress, cold exposure, and cigarette smoking. The foregoing findings suggest that dynamic changes in coronary artery size may play an important role in the pathogenesis of ischemia.

In addition, continuous electrocardiographic monitoring in both the coronary care unit and ambulatory setting, indicate that heart rate increases during the actual silent ischemic episode. This rise in heart rate appears, in part, to be mediated by $beta_1$ adrenergic activity, and would be expected to increase myocardial oxygen demands and limit time for diastolic coronary blood flow.

Therefore, this heart rate increase should increase the magnitude and duration of an ischemic episode. Frequent and prolonged episodes of silent ischemia at low heart rates, as seen in unstable angina patients, can identify a patient subset at high risk for coronary events (eg, recurrent unstable angina, myocardial infarction, sudden death) and may be a marker for coronary endothelial dysfunction. In contrast, patients with ischemia occurring only at high heart rates, seen during high level exercise tests, appear to be at low risk for events and may serve as a marker for normal endothelial function.

SUMMARY AND CONCLUSION

Recognition of the concept of silent ischemia as equivalent to a transient inadequacy in myocardial blood flow has led to a more complete understanding of the mechanisms of ischemia. The data suggest that a single pathophysiological mechanism is unlikely in any given patient, but must relate to both myocardial supply and demand factors. A consideration of these mechanisms and their management will lead to a more rational approach to altering the morbidity and mortality of ischemic heart disease than is found when considering pain alone.

BIBLIOGRAPHY

Bonow RO, Kent KM, Rosing DR, Lan KKG, Lakatos E, Borer JS, Bacharach SL, Green MV, Epstein SE. Exercise induced ischemia in mildly symptomatic patients with coronary artery disease and preserved left ventricular function. N Engl J Med 1984;311:1339-1345.

Chierchia S, Lazzari M, Freedman B, Brunelli C, Maseri A. Impairment of myocardial perfusion and function during painless myocardial ischemia. J Am Coll Cardiol 1983;1:924-930.

Cohn PF, Braunwald E. Chronic ischemic heart disease. In: Braunwald E, ed. Heart Disease: A Textbook Of Cardiovascular Medicine. Philadelphia: W. B. Saunders Co., 1984;1334-1383.

Coy K, Imperi G, Pepine CJ. Silent ischemia during daily activities in patients with asymptomatic positive exercise tests. Am J Cardiol 1987;59:45-49.

Curry RC, Pepine CJ, Conti CR. Ambulatory monitoring to evaluate therapy results in variant angina patients. (abstract) Circulation 1979;60:II-190.

Deanfield JE, Shea M, Ribiero P, De Landsheere CM, Wilson RA, Horlock P, Selwyn AP. Transient ST segment depression as a marker of myocardial ischemia during daily life. Am J Cardiol 1984;54:1195-1200.

Deanfield JE, Maseri A, Selwyn AP, Chierchia S, Riberio P, Krinkler S. Myocardial ischemia during daily life in patients with stable angina: its relation to symptoms and heart rate changes. Lancet 1983;2:753-758.

Droste C, Roskamm H. Experimental pain measurement in patients with asymptomatic myocardial ischemia. J Am Coll Cardiol 1983;1:940-945.

Ellestad MH, Wan MKC. Predictive implications of stress testing: follow up of 2700 subjects after maximum treadmill stress testing. Circulation 1975;51:363-369.

Erikssen J, Thaulow E. Follow-up of patients with asymptomatic myocardial ischemia. In: Rutishauser W, Roskamm H, ed. Silent Myocardial Ischemia. Berlin: Springer-Verlag, 1984;154-164.

Fuster V, Frye RL, Connolly DC, Danielson MA, Elveback LR, Kurland LT. Arteriographic patterns early in the onset of the coronary syndromes. Br Heart J 1975;37:1250.

Gottlieb SO, Weisfeldt ML, Ouyang P, Mellits ED, Gerstenblith G. Silent ischemia as a marker for early unfavorable outcomes in patients with unstable angina. N Engl J Med 1986;314:1214-1219.

Gottlieb SO, Ouyang P, Mellits ED, Gerstenblith G. Silent ischemia during medical therapy predicts unfavorable outcomes in unstable angina. N Engl J Med 1986;19:1214-1219.

Hultgren W, Peduzzi P, Pierpont G. Symptom severity and prognosis. Prog Cardiovasc Dis 1986;28:273-278.

Imperi GA, Lambert CR, Coy K, Lopez L, Pepine CJ. Effects of titrated beta blockade (metoprolol) on silent myocardial ischemia in ambulatory patients with coronary artery disease. Am J Cardiol 1987;60:519-524.

Johnson SM, Mauritson DR, Winniford MD, Willerson JR, Firth BG, Cary J, Hillis LD. Continuous electrocardiographic monitoring in patients with unstable angina pectoris: identification of high-risk subgroup with severe coronary disease, variant angina, and/or impaired early prognosis. Am Heart J 1982;103:4-12.

Lambert CR, Imperi GA, Pepine CJ. Low frequency requirements for recording ischemic ST segment abnormalities in man. Am J Cardiol 1986;58:225-229.

Leaman DM, Brower RW, Meester GT, Serruys P, Van den Brand M. Coronary artery atherosclerosis: severity of the disease, severity of angina pectoris and compromised left ventricular function. Circulation 1981;63:285.

Ludmer PL, Selwyn AP, Wayne RR, Mudge GM, Alexander RW, Ganz P. Impaired endothelial-dependent coronary dilation in patients with coronary artery disease. N Engl J Med 1986;315:1045.

Pepine CJ. Clinical aspects of silent myocardial ischemia in patients with angina and other forms of coronary heart disease. Am J Med 1986;80:25-34.

Proudfit WL, Shirey EK, Sones FM. Selective cine coronary arteriography: correlatin with clinical findings in 1000 patients. Circulation 1966;33:901.

Quyyumi AA, Wright CM, Mockus LJ, Fox KM. How important is a history of chest pain in determining the degree of ischemia in patients with angina pectoris? Br Heart J 1985;54:22-26.

Rocco MB, Barry J, Campbell S, Nabel EG, Rebecca GS, Selwyn AP. Circadian variation of transient myocardial ischemia. (abstract) J Am Coll Cardiol 1986;7:191A.

Schang SJ, Pepinc CJ. Transient asymptomatic ST segment depression during daily activity. Am J Cardiol 1977;39:396-402.

Selwyn AP, Fox K, Eves M, Oakley D, Dargie H, Shillingford J. Myocardial ischaemia in patients with frequent angina pectoris. Br

Med J 1978;2:1594-1596.

Selwyn AP, Allan R, L'Abbate A, Horlock P, Camici P, Clark J, O'Brien HA, Grant PM. Relationship between regional myocardial uptake of rubidium-82 and perfusion: absolute reduction of cation uptake in ischemia. Am J Cardiol 1982;50:112.

Sobel BE, Braunwald E. Coronary blood flow and myocarial ischemia. In: Braunwald E, ed. Herat Disease: A Textbook Of Cardiovascular Medicine. Philadelphia: W. B. Saunders Co., 1984;1234-1261.

Stern S, Tzivoni D. Early detection of silent ischemic heart disease by 24-hour electrocardiographic monitoring of active subjects. Br Heart J 1974;36:481-486.

Warnes CA, Roberts WC. Sudden coronary death: relation of amount and distribution of coronary narrowing at necropsy to previous symptoms of myocardial ischemia, left ventricular scarring and heart weight. Am J Cardiol 1984;54:65.

Weiner DA, Ryan TJ, McCabe CH, Chaitman BR, Sheffield LT, Ferguson JC, Fisher LD, Tristani F. Prognostic importance of a clinical profile and exercise test in medically treated patients with coronary artery disease. J Am Coll Cardiol 1984;3:772-779.

3

MYOCARDIAL ISCHEMIA AS A USEFUL FUNCTIONAL INDICATOR OF RISK IN PATIENTS WITH CORONARY ARTERY DISEASE

Andrew P. Selwyn, M.D., Khether Raby, Joan Barry, Michael B. Rocco, Kimberely Meade, Charles Treasure

The general problem of coronary disease It is generally true that obstructive coronary artery disease is the leading cause of disabling symptoms, heart failure and premature death in this country. Although medications, angioplasty and coronary surgery are widely used to help symptoms and reverse acute and high risk clinical syndromes, the disease still presents with many unheralded and damaging events. What is the evidence that most of the damaging pathology of obstructive coronary disease develops and presents without any symptoms or prior warning?

Sudden death in men and woman over the age of 45 years is a public health problem and the majority, by far, have obstructive coronary artery disease with some evidence of ischemic damage to the left ventricular myocardium. Patchy macroscopic scars that disturb LV function are commonly found at post mortem examination in older patients with developed 3 vessel coronary artery disease. One quarter to one third of myocardial infarcts occur in the community without diagnosis, or admission to the hospital and this event adversely effects prognosis while clinicians have known for years that signs of transient myocardial ischemia in patients with coronary artery disease can manifest without chest pain. Krayenbuhl and colleagues have shown that the functional disturbances of the left ventricle during transient ischemia without pain is equal in every way to the ischemia that effects the left ventricle with angina and studies of ischemic disturbances in myocardial perfusion have shown transient abnormalities during asymptomatic ischemia that are identical to those seen during chest pain. All of the above evidence would suggest that obstructive coronary disease will transiently deprive the left ventricle of its blood supply and that this basic pathophysiologic mechanism is the means by which the atherosclerosis finally damages left ventricular function causing symptoms, disability and death.

Clinical detection of ischemic heart disease

Epidemiological studies have identified risk factors that are used to assess the pre-test likelihood of coronary artery disease, but they lack precision in individual patients. As a result, non-invasive tests have been developed and use the electrocardiogram and radioisotopes during exercise, pacing or drugs, to provoke evidence of transient myocardial ischemia. These clinically useful techniques include exercise electrocardiography, stress thallium scintigraphy, radionuclide ventriculography with exercise, and finally, continuous monitoring of the electrocardiogram in ambulant patients. Rather than try and use these techniques for the detection of anatomical coronary disease, current research has emphasized that the evidence regarding the presence and severity of transient myocardial ischemia and its effect upon the left ventricle, provides an important assessment of the risk of future adverse coronary events. Therefore, the need of further testing, therapy and interventions can be determined. This review will discuss the application of these techniques and the emerging importance of ischemia as a clinical finding in and of itself when trying to protect patients against the damaging effects of obstructive coronary disease.

Sensitivity and specificity of tests for ischemia and risk: All of the tests that have been listed above should probably not be use in young people (under age 40) who present with few or no risk factors for coronary artery disease. One exception might include young individuals who present with typical angina pectoris. However, mass screening of the population is not justified at present because of the poor sensitivity and specificity in people with low pretest likelihood of coronary artery disease. However, the opposite is true in patients who are over 40 years of age who have one or more of the cardinal risk factors and may present with symptoms or concerns about heart disease. In these people, a technically satisfactory and negative test is extremely useful in reassuring the patient about the very low risk of adverse coronary events. Similarily, a positive test at a very high workload is accompanied by a good prognosis and could be followed by reassurance. However, clinical trials have demonstrated that an obviously positive test in this particular age group with risk factors, is a very important indicator being sensitive and specific for the detection of ischemia, and by inference, coronary artery disease. Each of the tests that are listed above have specific features that need attention in order to avoid lack of specificity and false positive results. This information has been extensively reviewed for the practicing clinician. For this review, it is reasonable to conclude that in patients over the age of 40 with one or more of the cardinal risk factors for coronary artery disease, these tests become sufficiently specific and sensitive to be useful in trying to detect ischemia as a functional marker of risk.

Variability: Variability of standardized exercise testing is not a major problem in the clinical application of this test, although there are considerable problems if the protocol is not standardized, or if for example, the test is done at different times of the day. The standardization of thallium scintigraphy and radionuclide ventriculography with normal values and quantitative results is still not generally available and the results are greatly effected by intrepretation. Finally, continuous monitoring of the electrocardiogram in ambulant patients outside of the hospital, is a convenient technique that has demonstrated frequent ischemia during daily life. Although this has uncovered many new characteristics of ischemic heart disease activity, the prolonged recording of this biological signal demonstrates considerable variability. Two studies have established that this can be understood for individuals and for groups of patients permitting a clear interpretation of the extent of increase or decrease in ischemic activity during daily life that is important and extends beyond the natural variability in stable patients.

Prognosis: There is ample evidence that a positive exercise test with evidence of ischemia, and particularly with a limited duration of exercise identifies subgroups at increased risk of coronary events. This has been true in totally asymptomatic men and women over the age of 45 years. It is also true in patients with angina pectoris, after myocardial infarction and following unstable angina pectoris. Studies using thallium scintigraphy and radionuclide ventriculography have also demonstrated the same results, that the number and extent of perfusion defects or the degree of disturbance of ejection fraction during exercise are potent indicators of the future risk of adverse coronary events providing independent information that is very useful. Information is now available that the quantitation of ischemia during continuous monitoring of the electrocardiogram while patients are ambulant out of hospital provides very similar results to the tests listed above. Again, active ischemia in stable patients identifies a group who are at increased risk of coronary events, whereas freedom from ischemia over 48-hours of monitoring appears to indicate a very low indicence of adverse coronary events.

It is of interest that all of the techniques listed above have different features, sources of error, levels of variability and technical demands, yet the studies have all produced the same results showing that the presence and severity of active transient ischemia affects prognosis. This indication of increased risk applies even when the patients are quite asymptomatic. It also applies in a wide variety of clinical presentations of coronary artery disease.

Treatment: The first order of clinical medicine is to relieve unpleasant symptoms and therefore the effective treatment of angina pectoris with reassurance is the first step in the management of patients. On the other hand, most clinicians will also seek evidence that there has been an objective improvement in the manifestation of disease. In this way, treatment is used in an attempt to improve signs that shift patients into a low risk clinical state. A wide range of commonly used therapuetic approaches are not applied with the full historic evidence of well-controlled clinical trials showing improved outcome. Indeed, many are used with the rational notion that they improve the measured evidence of disease activity and result in the objective improvement in the high risk manifestations of disease. This guiding principal is important if we consider that the relief of symptoms is necessary but insufficient and in the absence of absolute proof from pragmatic-controlled clinical trials, the clinician needs to make some attempt to diminish the risk of future adverse events. Finally, there is evidence that medical treatment, angioplasty and coronary surgery can certainly relieve pain, and they can also improve the evidence of ischemia on exercise testing, thallium scintigraphy and radionuclide ventriculography. Similarily, there are published trials to show that medical therapy, angioplasty and bypass surgery can produce significant improvement in the number and duration of ischemic episodes recorded during continuous monitoring of the electrocardiogram during daily life. Indeed, there is evidence from the Cass study that coronary surgery produces important improvements in mortality when used in patients who have 3-vessel coronary disease with evidence of active ischemia, whereas it appears to produce no such benefit in those patients who only have 3-vessel disease but no evidence of active ischemia.

Conclusions: There is abundant evidence that the damaging effects of obstructive coronary artery disease include transient ischemia, necrosis and progressive destruction of left ventricular function. Along with this evidence is the fact that most of this pathology can occur without any symptoms until the very last moments of disease manifestation. It appears to be quite wrong to consider ischemia only if it is associated with chest pain. A number of powerful clinical tests have been developed that can identify transient ischemia as a functional indicator of developing obstructive coronary disease and clinical trials have already shown that those patients with coronary disease who have active ischemia are at greatly increased risk of adverse coronary events whereas those with no active ischemia have a very good outcome by comparison. Clearly, there are a number of national clinical trials that address the issue of relief of obstructive coronary disease and active ischemia, morbidity and mortality. However, the clinician has to respond to three guiding principals in the present day management of patients with this disease. First, it is necessary to relieve symptoms. Next, it is necessary to assess the risk and dangers of future adverse coronary events and institute therapy that will tend to decrease these risks and move patients from higher risk to lower risk categories. Finally, practitioners must keep a very critical eye on prospective controlled clinical studies that demonstrate that the therapies that improve the objective manifestations of disease, do in fact result in diminished morbidity and mortality. The reality is that it is not always possible to utilize all three principals in the treatment of each patient, particularly during the life-long management of a disease that is imcompletely understood. Nevertheless, practice must continue along these guidelines as far as possible, as long as the remedies do not carry greater risks than the disease state.

REFERENCES

1. Nabel, E.G., Rocco, M.B., Barry, J., Campbell, S., and Selwyn, A.P. JAMA 257:1923-1928, 1987.

4

THE DIAGNOSTIC AND PROGNOSTIC VALUE OF EXERCISE ECG AND RADIONUCLIDE MARKERS OF ISCHEMIA IN ASYMPTOMATIC AND SYMPTOMATIC POPULATIONS

Robert S. Gibson, M. D.

INTRODUCTION

The concept of episodic myocardial ischemia occurring in the absence of symptoms has been appreciated for decades. In the past few years, however, this phenomena which has acquired the label "silent ischemia" has become a popular clinical concern among cardiologists and primary care physicians.[1-3] Despite great interest and much research in the area, a number of important issues remain unresolved.[4-5] These include: 1) What is the best method for detecting myocardial ischemia in various subgroups of patients with suspected or known CAD?; 2) is asymptomatic ischemia (versus no ischemia) associated with increased patient risk, and is the risk of major cardiovascular morbidity and mortality comparable to that observed in patients with symptomatic ischemia?; 3) do patients with asymptomatic ischemia have an abnormally high pain perception threshold, or simply less extensive CAD and a smaller ischemic burden than patients with symptomatic ischemia?; and, 4) what are the benefits of treating asymptomatic ischemia and should the established treatment for symptomatic patients including PCTA and coronary artery bypass surgery be applied to asymptomatic patients?.

Central to our understanding of silent ischemia, especially its prevalence, prognostic significance and response to treatment, is knowledge of the effectiveness of the technologies used to detect it.[5] Unfortunately, there is at present no widely available "gold standard" to validate the accuracy of noninvasive tests to define myocardial ischemia per se. If, however, we assume a linear relationship between the presence/extent of ischemia and the risk of future coronary events, the reliability of various noninvasive markers of ischemia can be compared. Accordingly, the purpose of this discussion is to examine whether or not the occurrence of specific cardiac events is accurately predicted by techniques commonly employed for the detection of silent ischemia - namely, exercise electrocardiography and thallium-201 (TL-201) myocardial perfusion scintigraphy.

Exercise Electrocardiography

Identification of myocardial ischemia has traditionally been based on the development of characteristic ST segment depression of at least 1.0 mm 80 msec after the J-point. The accuracy of this "characteristic" response, however, depends not only on the sensitivity and specificity of the ECG response, but also on the prevalence of CAD in the population being tested. According to Bayes' theorem,[6,7] we would expect that the predictive value of exercise-induced ST segment depression would be relatively high when observed in individuals with known, or strongly suspected CAD, but very low in asymptomatic, apparently healthy subjects.

Asymptomatic subjects. Exercise testing has been used to evaluate asymptomatic individuals in whom sudden incapacitation due to myocardial ischemia or infarction could compromise public safety. Such individuals include those engaged in hazardous occupations such as military or commercial aviation, firemen and policemen. The possibility of important asymptomatic ischemia is also of potential clinical concern among railroad engineers, air traffic controllers, and drivers of large commercial vehicles. Finally, because an unsupervised exercise program does present some risk to a sedentary, coronary-prone middle aged man, some physicians consider it prudent to evaluate such individuals with exercise testing before prescribing a vigorous exercise program.

Since myocardial ischemia is closely linked to the presence of large vessel CAD, it seems worthwhile to review the accuracy of exercise-induced ST segment depression for predicting significant angiographic disease (i.e., at least one major epicardial vessel with $\geq$ 50% stenosis). As shown in Table 1, when data from three studies[8-10] comprising 336 asymptomatic middle-aged men are pooled, the predictive value of a positive exercise test was only 26% (range 21 to 37%). Thus, in asymptomatic individuals, most abnormal ST segment responses are not related to CAD. The rather obvious implication of this finding is that a positive test, in the absence of chest pain, should not be used to predict the presence of angiographically significant CAD.

TABLE1. PREDICTIVE VALUE OF EXERCISE-INDUCED ST SEGMENT DEPRESSION FOR ANGIOGRAPHIC CAD IN ASYMPTOMATIC MEN

Study (year)	No. Pts. with positive exercise test	No. Pts. (%) with significant CAD
Borer (1975)	30	11 (37%)
Froelicher (1976)	111	34 (31%)
Uhl (1981)	195	41 (21%)
Pooled data	336	86 (26%)

Although a positive exercise test in an asymptomatic individual cannot be considered diagnostic of CAD, it does seem to indicate an increased risk of developing some clinical manifestation of CAD in the future. Table 2 summarizes seven epidemiologic studies[11–17] that have utilized maximal or near-maximal exercise testing to screen asymptomatic subjects for latent CAD. The populations in these studies were tested and followed for a mean of 3 to 12.7 years. During follow-up, the incidence of "clinical CAD" (i.e., angina pectoris, myocardial infarction [MI] and cardiac death) was recorded. When data from all 7 studies are pooled, one finds that the risk of developing one or more of the CAD endpoints was 4.2-times greater among patients with exercise-induced ST segment depression.

TABLE 2. PREDICTIVE VALUE OF EXERCISE-INDUCED ST SEGMENT DEPRESSION FOR THE DEVELOPEMENT OF CLINICAL CAD IN ASYMPTOMATIC SUBJECTS

Study (year)	Total No. Pts.	Follow-up years	Pts.(%) with events*	Event Rate by Group		Risk Ratio
				ST↓	No ST↓	
Froelicher (1974)	710	6.3	7(1.0%)	10.5%	0.7%	14.5
Cummings (1975)	510	3.0	26(5.1%)	24.6%	2.4%	10.3
Bruce (1980)	2365	5.6	47(2.0%)	5.3%	1.6%	3.3
Allen (1980)	888	5.0	48(5.4%)	14.4%	4.2%	3.4
MacIntyre (1981)	548	8.0	38(6.9%)	26.0%	6.1%	4.3
Giagnoni (1983)	514	6.0	34(6.6%)	15.6%	3.4%	4.5
McHenry (1984)	916	12.7	64(7.0%)	39.1%	6.3%	5.7
			Pooled Data	13.0%	3.1%	4.2

$$\text{Risk Ratio} = \frac{\text{\% with abnormal test who developed clinical CAD}}{\text{\% with normal test who developed clinical CAD}}$$

* Events include angina pectoris, MI or cardiac death

The data in Table 2 has sometimes been used to support the practice of screening asymptomatic subjects for latent CAD. Before endorsing a test strategy which uses exercise ST segment depression alone to identify a high-risk group, the physician should keep in mind the following points. First, only 13% of the subjects in Table 2 with a positive test had a coronary event during long-term follow-up. Since the vast majority of subjects (i.e., 87%) remained active and free of any clinical manifestation of CAD, a single positive exercise test should not necessarily be construed as a harbinger of future cardiovascular morbidity or mortality. Second, a positive exercise ECG in an asymptomatic individual has not been shown to predict increased risk of clinical CAD in men less than 40 years of age, women of any age, or in subjects without cardiac risk factors. Third, the Seattle Heart Watch Study[13] found that the likelihood of a subsequent coronary event was significantly increased only if ST segment depression was associated with exercise duration $\leq$ 6 minutes, chest pain or impaired heart rate response (i.e., failure to attain at least 90% of age predicted maximum heart rate). Finally, the study by McHenry et al[17] indicates that an abnormal ST segment response, while predictive of future angina, is not associated with an increased risk of death or MI as an initial event (Table 3). This last observation deserves considerable emphasis - as does the finding that the vast majority of deaths and nonfatal infarctions (33 of 34 [97%]) occurred in subjects with no ST segment depression.

TABLE 3. PREDICTIVE VALUE OF EXERCISE ECG FOR THE DEVELOPMENT OF SPECIFIC CARDIAC EVENTS IN ASYMPTOMATIC MIDDLE-AGED MEN*

Initial Event	No. Pts.(%) with event		Risk Ratio
	ST↓(n=23)	No ST↓(n=871)	
Angina pectoris (n=30)	8(34.8%)	22(2.5%)	13.8
Death or MI (n=34)	1(4.3%)	33(3.8%)	1.1

* During mean follow-up of 12.7 years

<u>Stable symptomatic patients</u>. Exercise testing is frequently used in symptomatic patients to determine whether or not chest pain is due to CAD. Since 1967, at least 16 studies comprising 5315 patients have correlated the presence of 1.0 mm or more of ST segment depression during maximal or near maximal exercise testing with coronary angiography.[7] The overall sensitivity of the test in these studies was 64% (range 47 to 81%). An important corollary of this average sensitivity value is the observation that 36% of patients with angiographically demonstrable CAD had negative ECG responses to exercise. Because of this high false negative rate among symptomatic patients referred for chest pain evaluation, the reliability of the stress electrocardiogram as a single test for detecting CAD has been seriously questioned.

Patients with known or strongly suspected CAD (i.e., those with documented angiographic stenoses, typical angina or previous infarction) sometimes undergo exercise testing for prognostic purposes. In this application, stress testing is performed to identify the group with high-risk coronary anatomy in whom aggressive management (e.g., PCTA or coronary bypass surgery) might be advisible because of evidence of severe reversible myocardial ischemia. The recent study by Podrid and colleagues[18], however, has placed some doubt on the use of exercise testing to identify such high-risk patients. In an effort to determine whether or not "profound" ST segment depression, irrespective of symptoms, is always associated with a poor prognosis, these investigators obtained follow-up on 142 medically-treated men with CAD who had reproducible 2.0 mm or more of ST segment depression during repeated treadmill examinations. The mean age of the study population was 57 years (range 39 to 80), 66% had a prior MI and 70% had exertional angina. Of interest, in 84 of the 142 patients (59%), the ST segment depression provoked by exercise was not associated with angina. During a mean follow-up of 5 years, only 10 patients (7.7%) died of cardiac causes (1.4% per year), 3 (2.1%) suffered MI (0.5%per year) and 9 patients (6.3%) required a myocardial revascularization procedure because of progressive angina (1.3% per year). The results of this study, at the very least, point out that it is necessary to consider variables other than the ECG response to exercise when attempting to identify patients at risk of major cardiovascular morbidity and mortality.

There is some evidence that the development of angina with exercise increases the likelihood that ST segment depression is due to prognostically important CAD.[13,19,20] In a study of 172 patients with 1.0 mm or more of ST segment depression, Weiner[19] found that both the presence and extent of atherosclerotic CAD (stenosis criteria $\geq$ 70%) was greater in patients with pain than in those without pain (Figure 1).

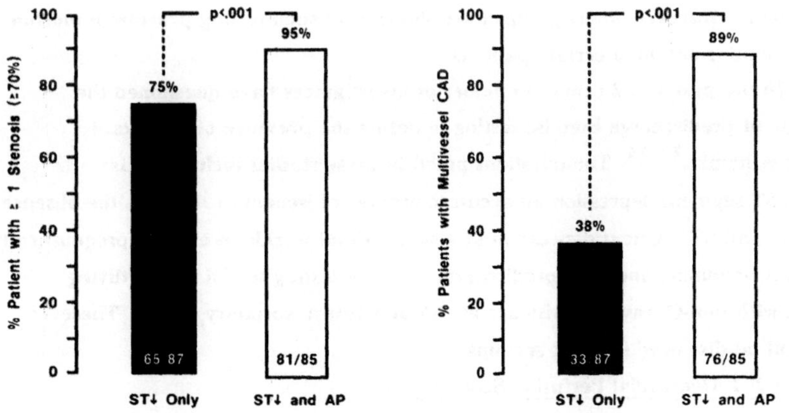

Figure 1. Predictive value of ST depression alone and ST depression with angina for CAD (left panel) and for multivessel CAD (right panel). Adapted from Weiner et al.[19]

Since patients with angina and ST depression appear to have more extensive underlying CAD than patients with ST depression alone, one might expect symptomatic ST depression to be associated with a less favorable prognosis. As shown in Figure 2, the findings of Cole and Ellestad[20] in 1402 patients who were followed for up to 7 years support this hypothesis.

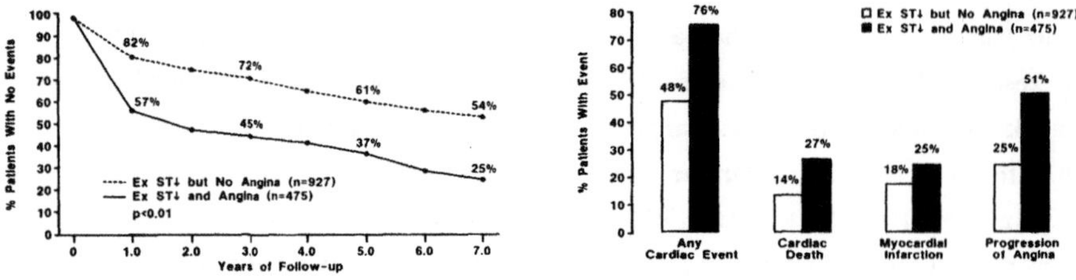

Figure 2. Prognosis of patients with ST depression alone versus ST depression with angina. Left panel illustrates probability of event-free survival. Right panel shows proportion of patients in each group with specific cardiac event. Adapted from Cole and Ellestad.[20]

<u>Patients with recent myocardial infarction.</u> The use of submaximal exercise testing in the assessment of patients recovering from acute uncomplicated MI has been the subject of extensive investigation during the past decade.[21] Its safety in selected patients and value in planning cardiac rehabilitation strategies are well established. Moreover, many groups have shown that such testing provides important prognostic information in certain patients.

In the past 1 to 2 years, a number of investigators have questioned the reliability of predischarge exercise testing to define the presence of important residual ischemia.[22-24] The questions posed in these studies include: 1) Is painless ST segment depression an accurate marker of ischemia? 2) Does the absence of angina and ST segment depression at a submaximal workload exclude prognostically important ischemia? and 3) Is predischarge exercise testing useful in identifying patients with non-Q-wave MI who are at risk of a future coronary event? These issues will be discussed in latter sections.

<u>Thallium-201 Myocardial Perfusion Scintigraphy</u>

Identification of myocardial ischemia by TL-201 scintigraphy is typically based on the demonstration of a transient perfusion abnormality[25] (Figure 3).

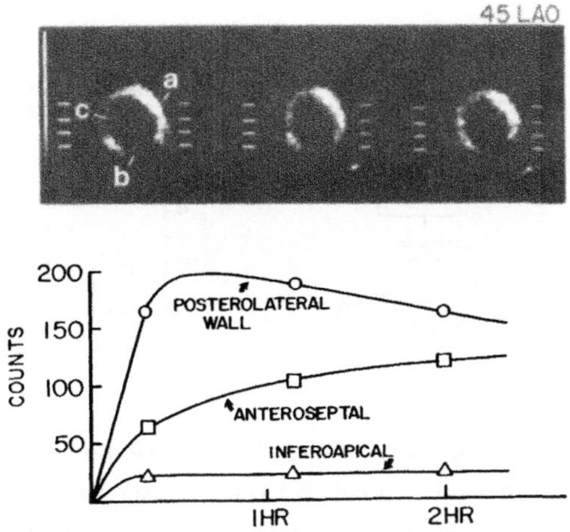

Figure 3. Sequential 45° LAO myocardial images (top) and the corresponding TL-201 time-activity curves in a patient with prior inferior myocardial infarction. The time-activity curves confirm normal uptake and washout of TL-201 in the postero-lateral segment (a), a persistent defect in the inferior apical segment (b) indicative of scar, and an initial defect with delayed redistribution in the anteroseptal segment (c) compatible with transient exercise-induced ischemia. Coronary angiography revealed a normal circumflex coronary artery, total occlusion of the right coronary artery and a 95% stenosis in the proximal anteiror descending coronary artery. From Gibson et al.[25]

<u>Asymptomatic subjects.</u> A number of investigators have evaluated the diagnostic value of TL-201 scintigraphy in asymptomatic subjects.[10,26-29] The largest study, by Uhl et al,[10] included 191 aircrewmen with positive exercise electrocardiograms. Of these, 135 had normal coronary angiographic findings, 15 had "subcritical" coronary stenosis (i.e., < 50% diameter narrowing) and 41 had significant CAD. As Figure 4 (left panel) shows, if the thallium scan was normal, the likelihood of disease was 1.4%, but it was 73.6% if thallium scintigraphic results were abnormal. These findings, which agree with other reports,[26-29] illustrate that while a positive stress ECG alone cannot be used to signify the presence of CAD (predictive value only 21.6%), the results of TL-201 scintigraphy can be used to sort out which subjects do not have significant CAD by angiographic criteria.

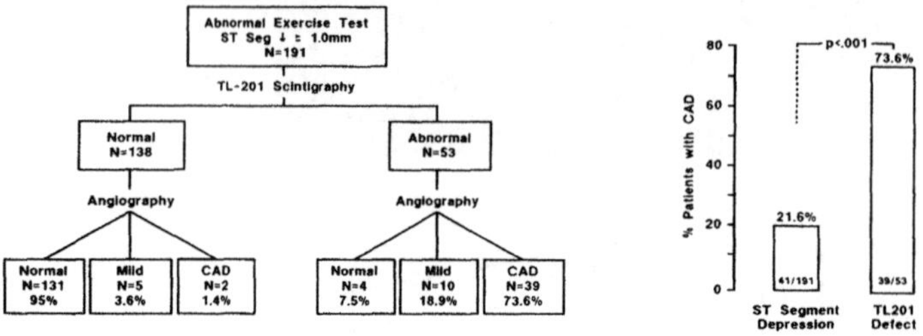

Figure 4. Thallium-201 and angiographic findings in 191 asymptomatic men with positive exercise ECG (left panel). The predictive value of exercise ST segment depression versus a TL-201 defect is shown in the right panel. Adapted from Uhl et al.[10]

Recently, Fleg and colleagues[30] from Baltimore reported preliminary data on the prognostic value of TL-201 scintigraphy in 34 clinically healthy volunteers (mean age 67 years) who had positive exercise tests by standard ECG criteria. During a mean follow-up of 2.9 years, 6 of the subjects (17.6%) experienced one or more cardiac events. When the outcome data was analyzed according to TL-201 results (i.e., presence or absence of focal perfusion abnormality), the incidence of a subsequent cardiac event was 7.1-times higher if scintigraphy was abnormal (5 of 14 [36%] versus 1 of 20 [5%] if normal). In light of these findings and those described above related to the diagnostic accuracy of TL-201 scintigraphy, it appears that the thallium stress test is more reliable than exercise electrocardiography for the detection of silent ischemia in the asymptomatic population.

Stable symptomatic patients. Many clinical studies have been published in which the sensitivity and specificity of TL-201 perfusion imaging were compared with the results of exercise ECG for detection of CAD in patients with chest pain. In one review of 2048 patients analyzed from 22 reports, the overall sensitivity and specificity of qualitative TL-201 scintigraphy (i.e., visual analysis of scintigraphic data) for CAD detection were 83% and 90%, respectively.[7] By comparison, the sensitivity and specificity of 1.0 mm or more of ischemic ST segment depression averaged 58% and 82%. When quantitative scan analysis of TL-201 myocardial uptake and washout are undertaken, both sensitivity and specificity approach 85 to 95%.[31-34]

Exercise TL-201 scintigraphy has been used effectively to stratify symptomatic patients into high- and low-risk categories.[35-40] Data from these studies indicate that the number of scan segments with abnormal TL-201 uptake on the initial post-exercise image, and the presence of delayed redistribution during sequential imaging (see Figure 3), are powerful predictors of subsequent ischemic cardiac events. Moreover, Brown and associates[35] from Boston have shown that the amount of myocardium at jeopardy for ischemia by TL-201 criteria is a better predictor of death or MI than either exercise ECG or the extent of CAD by angiography. This last observation should not be surprising as an abnormality on the thallium study reflects the pathophysiologic impact of CAD on nutrient blood flow reserve at the myocapillary level - which theoretically is of greater prognostic significance than mere delineation of the number of anatomic stenoses.

Several studies have indicated that patients with chest pain and a normal exercise TL-201 scintigram have an excellent prognosis even if angiographic CAD or exercise-induced ST segment depression has been demonstrated.[37-40] These reports which include between 95 and 455 symptomatic patients with follow-up ranging from 14 to 34 months show that the annual incidence of death and nonfatal MI is between 0-0.7% and 0.6-1.0%, respectively.

Patients with recent myocardial infarction. Detection of ischemia remote from the infarct zone (reflecting functionally significant multivessel CAD), residual ischemia within the infarct zone (common after non-Q-wave MI and in the post-thrombolytic patient), or both has been undertaken in patients with uncomplicated acute MI by means of predischarge stress testing and TL-201 scintigraphy.[22-24,41-48] Several groups have shown that perfusion defects in more than one specific vascular region is a more sensitive and accurate indicator of the presence of high-risk coronary anatomy (i.e., multivessel or left-main stem disease) than either ST segment depression or angina.[41-43,45]

Until recently, most physicians have assumed that exercise-induced ST-segment depression is a reliable marker of residual myocardial ischemia in patients recovering from an acute MI. While generally true for patients experiencing angina in conjunction with ST-segment depression, this conclusion no longer seems appropriate for those who have ST-segment depression alone. Indeed, in our experience,[22] fewer than 50% of patients with painless ST-segment depression during predischarge exercise ECG testing have evidence of ischemia by quantitative TL-201 scintigraphic criteria. These false-positive ECG responses are particularly common among patients with moderately large Q wave infarction resulting from occlusion of the RCA or left circumflex coronary arteries.

Does the absence of stress-induced angina and ST-segment depression (during submaximal exercise testing) exclude important residual ischemia? This issue was recently addressed by our group in 100 asymptomatic survivors of acute uncomplicated MI.[22] All patients had negative submaximal exercise tests a mean of 10 ± 3 days after onset of MI and each underwent quantitative TL-201 scintigraphy (in conjunction with the exercise test) and coronary angiography before discharge. A total of 44 patients (44%) were found to have multivessel CAD and the mean number of vessels with ≥ 50% stenoses for the entire group was 1.6 ± 0.8. Of interest, 49 of the 100 patients (49%) with negative exercise tests showed scintigraphic evidence of residual ischemia, either within the infarct zone or in myocardial segments remote from the zone of infarction. Moreover, when patients found to have ischemia on TL-201 testing were compared to those without ischemia, it was found that the former group had significantly greater mortality (10% vs 0%; $p < .05$) and a higher incidence of reinfarction (18% vs 2%; $p < .01$) during long-term follow-up. Indeed, the relative risk of experiencing either of these two "hard" cardiac events was 12 times greater (24% vs 2%; $p < .01$) among patients who demonstrated scintigraphic evidence of residual, albeit silent, ischemia. These results indicate that quantitative TL-201 perfusion imaging is a valuable adjunct to submaximal exercise testing, as its use can identify a large group of postinfarction patients with prognostically important ischemia who otherwise would not have been detected (Figure 5).

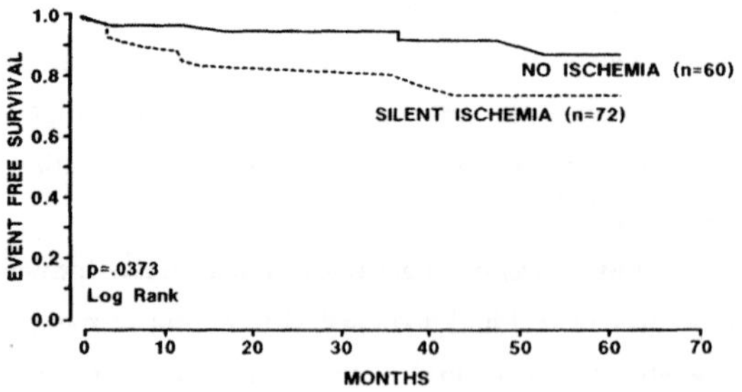

Figure 5. Kaplan-Meier survival curves for patients with no ischemia (solid line) and for patients with ischemia (dotted line) by exercise TL-201 scintigraphic criteria. All patients (n=132 as of 10/87) had negative submaximal exercise tests (i.e., no angina or ST depression) 10 ± 3 days after onset of MBCK confirmed acute MI. During long-term follow-up, the survival rate without reinfarction was significantly lower in patients with "silent ischemia" by TL-201 criteria (p=.0373 [Log rank]).

REFERENCES

1. Cohn JK, Cohn PF. Patient reactions to the diagnosis of asymptomatic coronary artery disease: implications for the primary physician and consultant cardiologist. J Am Coll Cardiol 1:956-958, 1983.
2. Singh BN (ed). Detection, quantification and clinical significance of silent myocardial ischemia in coronary artery disease (Symposium). Am J Cardiol 58:1B-60B, 1986.
3. Cohn PF, Kannel WB (eds). Recognition, pathogenesis and management options of silent coronary artery disease (Symposium). Circulation 75(Suppl 2):-1-54, 1987.
4. Kawanishi DT, Rahimtoola SH. Silent myocardial ischemia (Review with 197 references). Curr Probl Cardiol 12(9):511-566, 1987.
5. Berman DS, Rozanski A, Knoebel SB. The detection of silent ischemia: cautions and precautions (editorial). Circulation 75:101-106, 1987.
6. Diamond GA, Forrester JS, Hirsh M et al. Application of conditional probability analysis to the clinical diagnosis of coronary artery disease. J Clin Invest 65:1210-1221, 1980.
7. Gibson RS, Beller GA. Should exercise ECG testing be replaced by radionuclide methods? In Rahimtoola S, Brest A, eds.: Controversies in Coronary Artery Disease, Cardiovasc Clinics, Philadelphia, 1982, FA Davis, pp 1-31.
8. Borer JS, Brensike JF, Redwood DR et al. Limitations of the electrocardiographic response to exercise in predicting coronary artery disease. N Engl J Med 293:367, 1976.
9. Froelicher VF, Thompson AJ, Longo MR et al. Value of exercise testing for screening asymptomatic men for latent coronary artery disease. Prog Cardiovasc Dis 18:265-276, 1976.
10. Uhl GS, Kay TN, Hickman JR. Computer enhanced thallium scintigraphy in asymptomatic men with abnormal exercise 8:1037-1047, 1981.
11. Froelicher VF, Thomas MM, Pillow C et al. Epidemiologic study of asymptomatic men screened by maximal treadmill testing for latent coronary artery disease. Am J Cardiol 34:770-776, 1974.
12. Cummings GR, Samm J, Borysyk L et al. Electrocardiographic changes during exercise in asymptomatic men: 3-year follow-up. Can Med Assoc J 112:578-581, 1975.

13. Bruce RA, DeRouen TA, Hossack KF. Value of maximal exercise tests in risk assessment of primary coronary heart disease events in healthy men: Five years experience of the Seattle Heart Watch Study. Am J Cardiol 46:371-378, 1980.

14. Allen WH, Aronow WS, Goodman P et al. Five-year follow-up of maximal treadmill stress test in asymptomatic men and women. Circulation 62:522-527, 1980.

15. McIntyre NR, Kunkler JR, Mitchell RE et al. Eight-year follow-up of exercise electrocardiograms in healthy, middle-aged aviators. Aviat Space Envir Med 52:256-259, 1981.

16. Giagnoni E, Secchi MB, Wu SC et al. Prognostic value of exercise ECG testing in asymptomatic normotensive subjects: a prospective matched study. N Engl J Med 309:1085-1089, 1983.

17. McHenry PL, O'Donnell J, Morris SN et al. The abnormal exercise electrocardiogram in apparently healthy men: a predictor of angina pectoris as an initial coronary event during long-term follow-up. Circulation 70:547-551, 1984.

18. Podrid PJ, Graboys TB, Lown B. Prognosis of medically treated patients with coronary artery disease with profound ST segment depression during exercise testing. N Engl J Med 305:1111-1116, 1981.

19. Weiner DA, McCabe C, Hueter DC et al. Predictive value of chest pain as an indicator of coronary disease during stress testing. Am Heart J 96:458, 1978.

20. Cole JP, Ellestad MH. Significance of chest pain during treadmill exercise: correlation with coronary events. Am J Cardiol 41:227, 1978.

21. Froelicher VF, Perdue ST, Atwood JE et al. Exercise testing of patients recovering from myocardial infarction. Curr Probl Cardiol 11(7):370-444, 1986.

22. Gibson RS, Beller GA, Kaiser DL. Prevalence and clinical significance of painless ST segment depression during early postinfarction exercise testing. Circulation 75(Suppl 2):36-39, 1987.

23. Gibson RS. Detection and quantification of residual ischemia after acute uncomplicated myocardial infarction by thallium-201 scintigraphy. In Califf R, Mark D and Wagner GS (eds), Acute Coronary Care in the Thrombolytic Era. The Hague, Boston, Martinus-Nijhoff Publishers, 1987, in press.

24. Varma SK, Gibson RS. Predischarge exercise ECG versus thallium-201 in predicting prognosis after non-Q-wave myocardial infarction. Circulation, in press, 1987.

25. Gibson RS, Watson DD. Clinical applications of myocardial perfusion scintigraphy with thallium-201. In Yu P, Goodwin JE, eds.: Progress in Cardiology, Philadelphia, Lea and Febiger, 1984, pp 67-106.

26. Berman DS, Amsterdam EA, Joye JA et al. Thallium-201 stress myocardial scintigraphy: application in asymptomatic patients with positive exercise electrocardiograms. Am J Cardiol 41:380, 1978.

27. Caralis DG, Bailey I, Kennedy HL et al. Thallium-201 myocardial imaging in evaluation of asymptomatic individuals with ischemic ST segment depression on exercise electrocardiogram. Br Heart J 42:562-567, 1979.

28. Caralis DG, Bailey I, Kennedy HL et al. Screening asymptomatic middle aged men for obstructive coronary artery disease. Circulation 60(Suppl 2):149, 1979.

29. Guiney TE, Pohost GM, McKusick KA et al. Differentiation of false- from true-positive ECG responses to exercise stress by thallium-201 perfusion imaging. Chest 80:4-10, 1981.

30. Fleg JK, Gerstenblith G, Becker LC et al. Prognostic value of exercise electrocardiography and thallium scintigraphy in asymptomatic subjects. Circulation 68(Suppl 3):126, 1983.

31. Berger BC, Watson DD, Taylor GJ et al. Quantitative thallium-201 exercise scintigraphy for detection of coronary artery disease. J Nucl Med 22:585, 1981.

32. Maddahi J, Garcia EV, Berman DS et al. Improved noninvasive assessment of coronary artery disease by quantitative analysis of regional stress myocardial distribution and washout of thallium-201. Circulation 64:924, 1981.

33. Farris JV, Burt RW, Graham MC et al. Thallium-201 myocardial scintigraphy: improved sensitivity, specificity and predictive accuracy by application of a statistically image analysis algorithm. Am J Cardiol 49:733-742, 1982.

34. Wackers FJT, Fetterman RC, Mattero JA et al. Quantitative planar thallium-201 stress scintigraphy: a critical evaluation of the method. Sem Nucl Med 15:46, 1985.

35. Brown KA, Boucher CA, Okada RD et al. Prognostic value of exercise thallium-201 imaging in patients presenting for evaluation of chest pain. J Am Coll Cardiol 1:994-1001, 1983.

36. Ladenheim ML, Pollock BH, Rozanski A et al. Extent and severity of myocardial hypoperfusion as predictors of prognosis in patients with suspected coronary artery disease. J Am Coll Cardiol 7:464-471, 1986.

37. Staniloff H, Diamond G, Forrester J et al. Prediction of death, infarction and worsening chest pain with exercise electrocardiography and thallium scintigraphy. Am J Cardiol 49:957, 1982.

38. Pamelia FX, Gibson RS, Watson DD et al. Prognosis with chest pain and normal thallium-201 exercise scintigrams. Am J Cardiol 55:920-926, 1985.

39. Wackers FJT, Russo DJ, Russo D et al. Prognostic significance of normal quantitative planar thallium-201 stress scintigraphy in patients with chest pain. J Am Coll Cardiol 6:27-30, 1985.

40. Wahl J, Hakki AH, Iskandrian AS. Prognostic implications of normal exercise thallium-201 images. Arch Intern Med 145:253-256, 1985.

41. Dunn RF, Freedman B, Bailey IK et al. Noninvasive prediction of multivessel disease after myocardial infarction. Circulation 62:726, 1980.

42. Smeets JP, Rigo P, Legrand V et al. Prognostic value of thallium-201 stress myocardial scintigraphy with exercise ECG after myocardial infarction. Cardiol 68(Suppl 2):67-70, 1981.

43. Patterson RE, Horowitz SF, Eng C et al. Can noninvasive exercise test criteria identify patients with left main or 3-vessel coronary disease after a first myocardial infarction? Am J Cardiol 51:361-371, 1983.

44. Gibson RS, Watson DD, Craddock GB et al. Predicting cardiac events after uncomplicated acute myocardial infarction: a prospective study comparing predischarge exercise thallium-201 scintigraphy and coronary angiography. Circulation 68:321-336, 1983.

45. Gibson RS. The prognostic value of predischarge exercise thallium-201 scintigraphy after acute myocardial infarction. J Cardiovasc Rehab 5(1):28-39, 1985.

46. Leppo JA, O'Brien J, Rothender JA et al. Dipyridamole thallium-201 scintigraphy in the prediction of future cardiac events after acute myocardial infarction. N Engl J Med 310:1014-1018, 1984.

47. Melin JA, DeCoster PM, Renkin J et al. Effect of intracoronary thrombolytic therapy on exercise-induced ischemia after acute myocardial infarction. Am J Cardiol 56:705-711, 1985.

48. Gibson RS, Beller GA, Gheorghiade M et al. Prevalence and clinical significance of residual myocardial ischemia 2 weeks after uncomplicated non-Q-wave infarction: a prospective natural history study. Circulation 73:1186-1198, 1986.

5

AN INTEGRATED CLINICAL CLASSIFICATION FOR ISCHEMIC HEART DISEASE:

A COMBINED ASSESSMENT OF SEVERITY OF CORONARY DISEASE, LEFT VENTRICULAR FUNCTION AND MYOCARDIAL ISCHEMIA

Sidney O. Gottlieb, M.D.
Assistant Professor of Medicine
The Johns Hopkins University School of Medicine

INTRODUCTION

The traditional clinical classifications of patients with coronary heart disease have utilized either a descriptive categorization ot the extent of coronary artery disease, ie. single, double or triple vessel disease, or have relied on a description of the associated pattern of symptoms of angina pectoris. Although numerous studies have demonstrated the importance of the extent of disease and symptomatology in diagnosis and management (1-5), it is becoming increasingly clear that symptoms of angina may be poorly correlated with prognosis as angina may be an insensitive marker of the activity of ischemic heart disease (6-10). It is therefore important that the descriptive clinical classifications be revised by integrating the three major components influencing prognosis and management including coronary anatomy, left ventricular function, and the presence and extent of myocardial ischemia.

Coronary Artery Disease Severity

Studies have clearly demonstrated the importance of both the extent and distribution of coronary artery atherosclerotic obstructions in determining prognosis and guiding appropriate therapy (1-5). Although the extent of coronary disease is rather crudely assessed in terms of single, double or triple vessel disease with 50% or 70% diameter obstructions based on visual estimation of coronary angiograms, more sophisticated coronary disease assessments such as the Gensini Score (11) and others involving estimation of the percent of myocardium supplied by obstructed vessels (13) provide useful parameters to stratify patients into different risk groups. In addition, the severity of coronary disease has been shown to significantly influence the impact of various therapeutic interventions such as coronary bypass surgery, as patients with triple vessel disease with or without impaired left ventricular function have been shown to have improved survival with bypass surgical management compared to medical therapy (3,13,14). Also, surgical trials have demonstrated the importance of bypass surgery prolonging survival in subsets of patients with left main coronary artery disease (4). Although the knowledge of the number of diseased coronary arteries is important in determining risk in large clinical trials, this risk is clearly modified by other factors such as extent of left ventricular function and ongoing myocardial ischemia. In the CASS trial, for example, there was no difference in survival between those subsets of patients with triple vessel disease in the medical and surgical arm in the overall population (1), only when impaired left ventricular function was present could a difference be demonstrated (13). In addition, subset analysis has demonstrated that those with double vessel disease with objective evidence of myocardial ischemia on treadmill testing might also benefit with improved survival with bypass surgery (15), thus indicating that both left ventricular function and evidence of ongoing ischemia significantly modify the knowledge of coronary anatomy in assessing risk and appropriate treatment.

From a physiological standpoint, with the understanding of the importance of dynamic coronary obstructions mediated by vasoconstriction (16,17) and platelet aggregation and thrombosis (18-20), it is becoming clear that the presence of atherosclerotic obstructions by itself provides us with anatomic information which does not necessarily provide insight into the activity of the disease at the particular lesion sites which is of vital importance in assessing appropriate management.

Left Ventricular Function:

Studies have emphasized the importance of left ventricular function in determining risk in subsets with coronary artery disease (21,22). While patients with impaired left ventricular function, ie. left ventricular ejection fraction 40% or less, have a markedly increased mortality rate this knowledge by itself is again incomplete in assessing prognosis and appropriate management as patients with severe pre-infarction ischemic conditions may have normal left ventricular function but may nonetheless have extensive myocardium at risk (2). Clinical trials in unstable angina include patients with mostly normal resting left ventricular function, but nonetheless demonstrate the high risk of this condition (2,23). Therefore, an integration of the knowledge of left ventricular function with the extent of coronary disease and ongoing myocardial ischemia is important.

The knowledge of left ventricular function is particularly important to integrate with the knowledge of coronary artery disease severity as demonstrated by surgical trials in coronary disease. The CASS example as discussed above (1,13), and also the Veteran's Cooperative Unstable Angina Study (14) demonstrated the benefit or survival rates of surgery only in the subset of patients with impaired resting left ventricular function (LVEF <50%). The severity of left ventricular dysfunction may often co-vary with the severity of coronary artery disease, but this is not necessarily true in all cases, as patients with severe cardiomyopathy may have little atherosclerotic disease, and patients with extensive coronary disease may have normal left ventricular function.

Assessment of Myocardial Ischemia: Presence and Severity

Although traditional clinical classifications have relied upon the associated symptoms of myocardial ischemia, ie. stable or unstable angina, angina may be minimal or absent in many cases despite evidence of severe myocardial ischemia and extensive coronary artery disease. In addition, clinical studies have demonstrated that angina itself is a poor marker of prognosis or extent of disease (8-10, 24-26), whereas objective tests identifying myocardial ischemia such as exercise treadmill tests (27,29), radionuclide studies (30,31) and recently Holter monitoring (9,24-26) appear to be correlated with prognosis. Therefore, it appears important from a clinical point of view to focus our attention on the presence and severity of objective evidence for myocardial ischemia itself, which may or may not be associated with the symptom of angina pectoris in the management of our patients with this disease. The classification of "stable" or "unstable" should be based on objective evidence of ischemia rather than merely the angina pattern.

Significant insight into the presence and severity of myocardial ischemia is gained from exercise treadmill testing. This may identify the presence of coronary artery disease in asymptomatic populations where the presence of even silent myocardial ischemia has been demonstrated to predict an increased risk of mortality and non-fatal coronary events (27-29). The severity of ischemia may be assessed by the level at which an exercise test demonstrates ischemia, the duration of ischemia and the blood pressure response during exercise (32). In the early post infarction setting, the exercise test may indicate objective evidence of recurrent ischemia despite the fact that up to 50% of such individuals may be asymptomatic (10,33,34). Nevertheless, the presence of ischemia is independently associated with apparent prognosis following myocardial infarction and most agree that it should be aggressively treated. While the pattern of angina pectoris may clearly indicate increased risk and may significantly impact on the quality of life if it is frequent and persistent, we should continue to focus on this symptom ischemia <u>if it is present</u>. However, if we rely exclusively on angina, we will miss those patients who remain at high risk despite minimal or no symptoms.

Radionuclide studies using thallium 201 scintigraphy (31), gated blood pool scanning (36), and newer tomographic techniques (35) can significantly improve the diagnostic accuracy of exercise testing as they provide evidence of impairment of myocardial flow or transient left ventricular dysfunction. These tests may further provide diagnostic and prognostic information with objective evidence of ischemia.

Holter monitoring has been shown to be effective in patients with known coronary disease in detecting the presence and extent of episodes of ischemia occurring during normal daily life, which in many cases appear not to be provoked by marked increases in myocardial oxygen demands measured by heart rate and blood pressure (6,7). Studies in stable and unstable angina (9,24-26) and post-infarction patients (38) have recently suggested an impaired prognosis when Holter detected silent ischemia is present. Although most investigators agree that Holter monitoring is not presently an acceptable way of screening general populations for the presence of ischemic heart disease due to technical and interpretative difficulties, it appears to be useful to assess coronary disease activity by allowing for a greater window of observation in the out-of-hospital setting. This methodology provides another way to obtain objective evidence of myocardial ischemia to assess disease activity and prognosis.

An Integrated Clinical Classification for Ischemic Heart Disease:

It appears clear that we should abandon the older anatomic or symptomatic classifications of ischemic heart disease in favor of an integrated clinical approach involving the three cardinal prognostic variables: 1) extent of coronary artery disease, 2) left ventricular function, and 3) presence and severity of myocardial ischemia. In order to fully assess prognosis and management options, knowledge of all three is important. This is not to suggest that all patients must undergo testing to evaluate all three aspects, since several of the aspects may be interrelated and provide insight about each other.

The scheme identified in Table 1 and Figure 1 suggests a three-pronged classification. First, the presence and extent of coronary artery disease can be most simply stated as single, double, or triple vessel coronary artery disease and the presence of left main disease. Since the angiographically assessed extent of coronary disease may not fully reflect the true physiologic coronary flow abnormalities, it is not possible to state whether a lesion threshold of 50% or 70% diameter obstruction by visual or quantitative angiographic assessment is the most useful, however most clinical trials have utilized a 70% diameter obstruction threshold and this appears reasonable. Although further improvement of assessment may be obtained by such classifications as the Gensini Score (11) and percentage of myocardium supplied by significantly obstructed vessels (12), this is more specialized and complex and therefore may be more difficult to utilize in a general classification scheme for primary physicians as well as

TABLE I

1. Extent of Coronary Artery Disease ($\geq$ 70% diameter obstruction)

a. Left main

b. 1, 2, 3 vessel disease (proximal LAD, 2 vessel)

"% myocardium at risk"

2. Left Ventricular Function

a. LVEF < 40%, $\geq$ 40%

3. Presence and Severity of Myocardial Ischemia

a. Angina symptoms - none, stable, unstable

b. Recent (prior) infarction

c. Objective evidence of ischemia

i. Provocable: exercise treadmill test, thallium scintigraphy, exercise angiography

ii. "Spontaneous": Holter monitoring

EVALUATION OF PATIENTS WITH CORONARY DISEASE

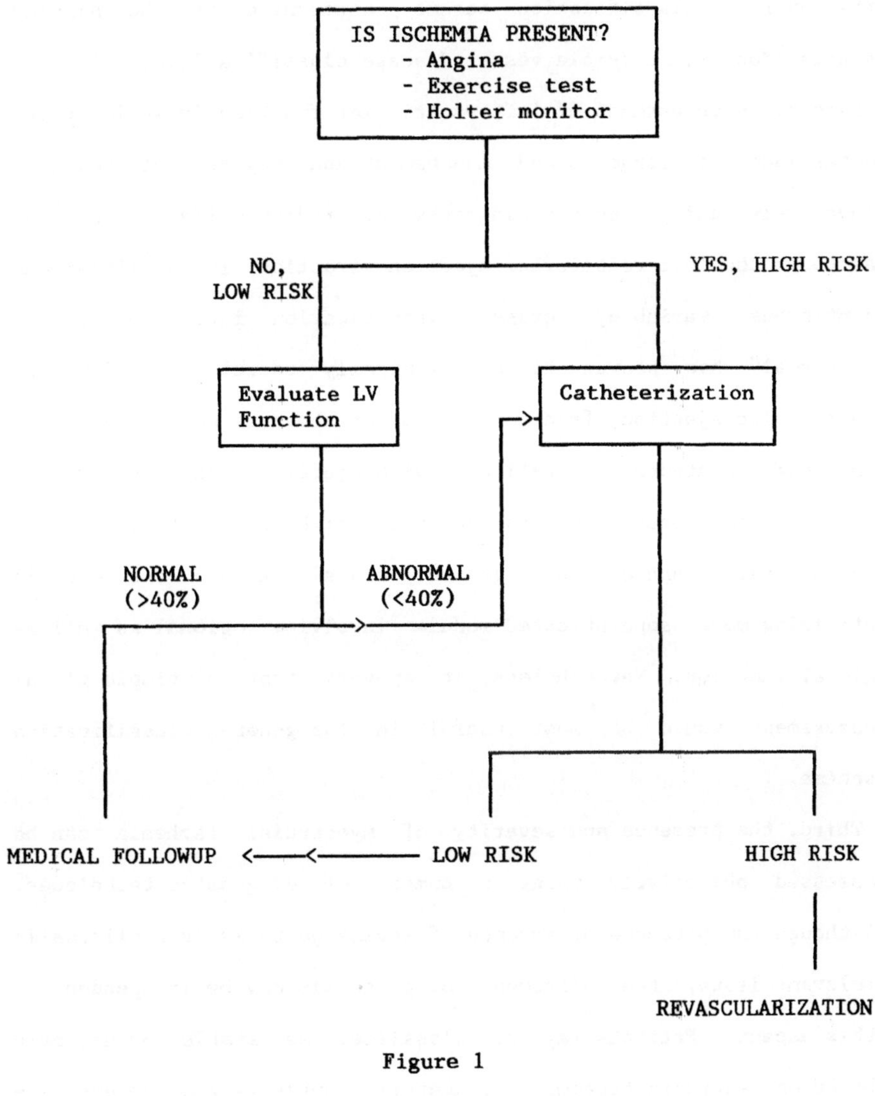

Figure 1

specialists. Also, the presence of complex and eccentric coronary stenoses may modify the risk as these appear to be more common in unstable angina patients (39), but this is another refinement of the overall classification scheme represented by the simpler single, double, or triple vessel disease classification.

Second, an assessment of left ventricular function is an important determinant of prognosis and management and may be obtained non-invasively using echocardiography or radionuclide techniques. Although the left ventricular ejection fraction is a linear and continuous variable, gross classification into "normal" or "abnormal" has proven to be clinically useful utilizing left ventricular ejection fraction of 45% or above as normal, and less than 45% as abnormal. Patients with ejection fractions of less than 35% have been found to be at the highest risk (40). Again, further refinement of this general classifications are possible utilizing more sophisticated models involving regional as well as global function. Nevertheless, it appears that a simple global assessment would be most useful in the general classification scheme.

Third, the presence and severity of myocardial ischemia can be assessed objectively using a number of diagnostic techniques. Although the presence or absence of angina pectoris is a clinically relevant issue, the assessment of prognosis may be independent of this aspect. Patients may be classified as stable or unstable based on exercise treadmill parameters; subjects who can exercise to six METS or above on standard exercise protocol without ischemia are at lower risk, whereas patients with early, global and severe evidence of myocardial ischemia with associated hemodynamic consequences such as drop in blood pressure are at highest risk. High risk parameters can also be identified using the more sophisticated methods such as thallium scintigraphy and radionuclide ventriculography during exercise and may also help to categorize patients into high and low risk. Although Holter monitoring has not been tested as extensively for risk assessment, it appears that frequent and prolonged periods of ischemia, ie. more than six episodes per 24 hours of ST depression or a cumulative duration of ischemia of greater than 60 minutes per 24 hours appears to identify higher risk patients (8,24). The extent to which the Holter data should modify the treadmill findings are unclear at this time and are under investigation. Again, the frequency and severity of angina is a clinically and prognostically useful variable when this is present and should be considered as part of the picture of evidence of ongoing myocardial ischemia, but only as part of the story as other objective and more reliable means of assessing this are also available.

Since these three general classification parameters may be interrelated, as patients with severe obstructive coronary disease often show evidence of myocardial ischemia in treadmill testing, it is not necessary to perform invasive procedures such as catheterization in all patients in order to classify them for clinical purposes. Since we know that patients without objective evidence of ischemia on treadmill testing and normal left ventricular function have a good overall prognosis, such patients would not undergo diagnostic angiography unless other modifying factors are present. However, some additional objective evidence of coronary artery disease should be sought to confirm the results of ST segment abnormalities on exercise testing such as thallium scintigraphy to make sure that exercise ST responses are not false positive or symptoms are not from another source such as gastrointestinal origin. However, since a plethora of medical regimens and interventional procedures such as coronary angioplasty and bypass surgery and thrombolytic therapy may be offered to selective subsets, knowledge of coronary anatomy in many cases is critical to implementation of these procedures and thus is an important part of assessment of risk and the decision process for appropriate management strategies.

SUMMARY

An integrated clinical classification for patients with coronary heart disease is presented which incorporates knowledge of coronary artery anatomy, left ventricular function, and presence and extent of provokable and spontaneous myocardial ischemia. Knowledge of information from each of these catagories may provide integrated prognostic and therapeutic information which we should utilize in communication regarding patients with this disorder. In addition, pathophysiologic and practical insights may be gained by seeking this information in a structured and organized fashion which may allow for a better understanding and management of patients with coronary heart disease.

REFERENCES

1. CASS Principle Investigators and Their Associates: Coronary Artery Sugery Study (CASS): A randomized trial of coronary artery bypass surgery. Survival data. Circulation 1983, 68:939.

2. Russell RO Jr., Moraski RE, Kouchoukos N, et al. Unstable angina pectoris: national cooperative study group to compare medical and surgical therapy. II. In-hospital experience and initial follow-up results in patients with one, two and three vessel disease. Amer J Cardiol 1978, 42:839-848

3. Taylor GJ, Humphries JO, Mellits ED, Pitt B, Schulze RA, Griffith LSC, Achuff SC. Predictors of clinical course, coronary anatomy and left ventricular function after recovery from acute myocardial infarction. Circulation 1980, 69:250-258.

4. Chaitman BR, Fisher LD, Bourassa MG, et al. Effect of coronary artery bypass surgery on survival patterns in subsets of patients with left main coronary artery disease. Report of the collaborative study in coronary artery surgery (CASS). Am J Cardiol 1981, 48:765.

5. Prospective randomized study of coronary artery bypass surgery in stable angina pectoris: second interim report by the European Coronary Surgery Study Group. Lancet 1980, 2:491-495.

6. Schang Jr. SJ, Pepine CJ. Transient asymptomatic ST segment derpression during daily activity. Am J Cardiol 1977, 39:396-400.

7. Deanfield J, Maseri A, Selwyn AP, et al. Myocardial ischemia during daily life in patients with stable angina: its relation to symptoms and heart rate changes. Lancet 1983, 2:753-758.

8. Hultgren. Symptom severity and prognosis. Prog in CV Dis 1986, 28:273-78.

9. Gottlieb SO, Weisfeldt R, Ouyang P, Mellits ED, Gerstenblith G. Silent ischemia as a marker for early unfarvorable outcomes in patients with unstable angina. N Engl J Med 1986, 314:1214-1219.

10. Weiner DA, Ryan TJ, McCabe CH, Luk S, Chaitman BR, Sheffield LT, Tristani F, Fisher LD. Significance of silent myocardial ischemia during exercise testing in patients with coronary artery disease. Am J Cardiol 1987, 59:725-29.

11. Gensini GG. Coronary arteriography. Mout Kisco, NY. Furtura Publishing Co. 31975, p. 261.

12. Ouyang P, Brinker JA, Mellits ED, Weisfeldt ML, Gerstenblith G. Variables predictive of successful medical therapy in patients with unstable angina: selection by multivariate analysis from clinical, electrocardiographic and angiographic evaluations. Circulation 1984, 70:367-376.

13. Passamani E, Davis KB, Gillespie MJ, Killip T, and the CASS principal investigators and their associates. A randomized trial of coronary artery bypass surgery: survival of patients with a low ejection fraction. N Engl J Med 1985, 312:1665-1671.

14. Luchi RJ, and the Veterans Administration Cooperative Study Group. Comparison of medical and surgical treatment for unstable angina pectoris. N Engl J Med 1987, 316:977-984.

15. Chaitman BR, Davis KB, et al. The role of coronary bypass surgery for "Left Main equivalent" coronary disease: The Coronary Artery Surgery STudy Registry. Cardiovascular surg 1985, Part 2. Circulation 1986, 74:S17.

16. Maseri A, L'Abbate A, Baroldi G, et al. Coronary vasospasm as a possible cause of myocardial infarction: a conclusion derived from the study of "preinfarction" angina. N Engl J Med 1978, 299:1271-1277.

17. Ludmer PL, Selwyn AP, Shook TL, et al. Paradoxical vasoconstriction induced by acetylcholine in atherosclerotic coronary arteries. N Engl J Med 1986; 315:1046-51.

18. DeWood MA, Spores J, Notske R, Mouser LT, Burroughs R, Golden MS, Lang HT. Prevalence of total coronary occlusion during the early hours of transmural myocardial infarction. N Engl J Med 1980, 303:897.

19. Sherman CT, Litvak F, Grundfest W, et al. Coronary angioscopy in patients with unstable angina pectoris. N Engl J Med 1986, 315:913-919.

20. Fitzgerald DJ, Roy L, Catella F, FitzGerald GA. platelet activation in unstable coronary disease. N Engl J Med 1986, 315:983-989.

21. The Multicenter Postinfarction Research Group. Risk stratification and survival after myocardial infarction. N Engl J Med 1983, 309:331-336.

22. Bigger JT, Fleiss JL, Kleiger R, Miller JP, Rolnitzky LM. The relationship among ventricular arrhythmias, left ventricular dysfunction, and mortality in the 2 years after

myocardial infarction. Circulation 1984, 69:250-258.

23. Gerstenblith G, Ouyang P, Achuff SC, et al. Nifedipine in unstable angina: a double-blind, randomized trial. N Engl J Med 1982, 306:885-9.

24. Nademanee K, Intarachot V, Josephson MA, Rieders D, Vaghaiwalla F, Singh BN. Prognostic significance of silent myocardial ischemia in patients with unstable angina. J Am Coll Cardiol 1987, 10:1-9.

25. Johnson SM, Mauritson DR, Winniford MD, et al. Continuous electrocardiographic monitoring in patients with unstable angina pectoris: identification of high-risk subgroup with severe coronary disease, variant angina and/or impaired early prognosis. Am Heart J 1982, 103:4-12.

26. Gottlieb SO, Weisfeldt ML, Ouyang P, Mellits ED, Gerstenblith G. Silent ischemia predicts infarction and death during 2 year follow-up of unstable angina. J Am Coll Cardiol 1987; 10:756-60.

27. Multiple Risk Factor Intervention Trial Research Group. Exercise electrocardiogram and coronary heart disease mortality in the multiple risk factor intervention trial. Am J Cardiol 1985, 55:16-24.

28. Giagnoni E, Secchi MB, Wu SC, Morabito A, Oltrona L, Mancarella S, Bolpin N, Fossal, Bettazzi L, Arangio G, Sachero A, Folli G. Prognostic value of exercise EKG testing in asymptomatic normotensive subjects: a prospective matched study. N Engl J med 1983, 309:1085-1088.

29. Gordon DJ, Ekelund LG, Karon JM, Probstfield JL, Rubenstien C, Sheffield LT, Weissfeld L. Predictive value of the exercise tolerance test for martality in North American men: the Lipid Research Clinics mortality follow-up study. Circulation 74 1986, 2:252-61.

30. Hung J, Goris, ML, Nash E, Kraemer HC, DeBusk RF, Berger III WE, Lew H. Comparative value of maximal treadmill testing, exercise thallium myocardial prefusion scintigraphy and exercise radionuclide ventriculography for distinguishing high- and low-risk patients soon after acute myocardial infarction. Am J Cardiol 1984, 53:1221-1227.

31. Gibson RS, Watson DD, Craddock GB, Crampton RS, Kaiser DL, Denny MJ, Beller GA. Prediction of cardiac events after uncomplicated myocardial infarction: a prospective study comparing predischarge exercise thallium-201 scintigraphy and coronary angiography. Circulaion 1983, 68:321-336.

32. McNeer JF, Margolis JR, Lee KL, Kisslo JA, Peter RH, Kong Y, Behar VS, Wallace AG, McCants CB, Rosati RA. The role of the exercise test in the evaluation of patients for ischemic heart disease. Circulation 1978, 57:64.

33. Theroux P, Waters DD, Halphen C, Debaisieux JC, Mizgala HF. Prognostic value of exercise testing soon after myocardial infarction. N Engl J Med 1979, 301:341-345.

34. Ouyang P, Shapiro EP, Chandra NC, Gottlieb SH, Chew PH, Gottlieb SO. An angiographic and functional comparison of patients with silent and symptomatic treadmill ischemia early after myocardial infarction. Am J Cardiol 1987, 59:730-734.

35. Nohara R, Kambara H, Suzuki Y, Tamaki S, Kadota K, Kawai C, Tamaki N, Torizuka K. Stress scintigraphy using single-photon emission computed tomography in the evaluation of coronary artery disease. Am J Cardiol 1984, 53:1250-54.

36. Borer J, Bacharach SL, Green MV, Kent KM, Epstein SE and Johnston GS. Real-time radionuclide cineangiorgraphy in the noninvasive evaluation of global and regional left ventricular function at rest and during exercise in patients with coronary artery disease. N Engl J Med 1977, 296:839-844.

37. Stern S, Tzivoni D. Early detection of silent ischaemic heart disease by 24-hour electrocardiographic monitoring of active subjects. Br Heart J 1974, 36:481-486.

38. Gottlieb SH, Gerstenblith G, Achuff SC, Mellits ED, Gottlieb SO. Ischemic ST segment changes by ambulatory Holter predict one year mortality in high risk postinfarct patients. Circulation 1986, 74(Suppl II):II-58.

39. Ambrose JA, Winters SL, Stern A, Eng A, Teichholz LE, Gorlin R, Fuster V. Angiographic morphology and the pathogenesis of unstable angina pectoris. J Am Coll Cardiol 1985, 5:609-619.

40. Schulze RA, Strauss HW, Pitt B. Sudden death in the year following myocardial infarction. Am J Med 1977, 62:192-199.

DISCUSSION - 1

Dr. Morganroth: Assume you saw a male patient who has high cholesterol and that he came to his physician you because his insurance man says he needs to have a treadmill test to qualify for a life insurance policy. You do a treadmill test and on it he has asymptomatic ST segment changes compatible with silent ischemia. What would you do next?

Dr. Cohn: I am sure that my colleagues do not recommend mass screening of all middle age males in this country looking for latent or silent heart disease. If someone walks into my office with a cholesterol of 250, is a cigarette smoker, has high blood pressure, and tells me his father dropped dead of a heart attack at age 50, I would be very foolish not to screen that individual for ischemia. Let's assume the stress test is positive. Now positive means different things to physicians. It is one of the major problems we have with stress testing in that it is interpreted as positive or negative. I will just give you an example. A stress test in which the patient goes for 15 minutes on the treadmill, has a very high heart rate and blood pressure product and has 1 mm of ST segment depression is considered positive. Also considered positive is the person who after 1 minute on the treadmill with a heart rate of 70, drops his ST segments by 5 mm without pain. These two tests examples are both considered positive but they have very very different meanings. Let's consider the patient with a positive exercise test at a very high work load. I would interpret that as of no clinical significance whatsoever. If he had a very positive one on the other hand at a lower work load and he came to us fortuitously because of this, I think we would be obligated to pursue this and the way that I would pursue this in a man with a positive test of some reasonableness, let's say 1 mm at 6 minutes, is to turn to my radionucleid colleagues and suggest that perhaps we should get a thallium test to make sure that exercise test was indeed positive. Suppose the positive thallium and ECG stress test is in a middle age male. That is the kind of individual where you have documented with high probability that there is some coronary disease present, you don't know how much, and you have two choices, just as if he had presented with mild angina. You could treat him, you could watch him with risk factor management, you could put him on an "anginal medication" which of course is an anti-ischemic, or you could study him and see the anatomy, (just as you could for patients if they presented with angina). If I was a practicing physician in an office, I would probably manage that patient rather conservatively. If I am in a University Hospital Center, in which I am trying to acquire more data on the natural history of these people, then I might do an angiogram. So it depends on the circumstance.

I would like to make one point to clarify what Dr. Pepine said in passing. When I proposed a defective anginal warning system to talk about the fact that these people don't have a warning, who are asymptomatic, it was not meant as a pathological kind of thing. In other words I don't think there is any discreet anatomical or neurological defect somewhere. I didn't mean it like that. I meant it as a clinical classification. For some reason they are not responding to the usual pain stimuli. I just wanted to clarify that point.

Dr. Morganroth: Do you have an explanation as to why?

Dr. Cohn: No, we don't have an explanation for why and some patients do have neurological defects, but others don't. It is a clinical classification.

Dr. Morganroth: Before we go on, I must ask you to define one word for us. You said for this supposed middle age, moderate high risk individual with cardiovascular risk factors in whom you find an abnormal ST segment response to exercise at low to medium level of exercise, you would move to a Thallium stress test. If the thallium test demonstrated reversal ischemia, you would treat him conservatively.

Dr. Cohn : It was perfectly all right to do that.

Dr. Morganroth: All right, I would like you to tell us what you mean by that, conservatively, is that with medicines?

Dr. Cohn: That could be with risk factor modification although in this man of course as you know, there is not much to modify. You could put him on a medication which would prolong his exercise tolerance. It depends. I personally don't believe it is a good thing for the heart to be rendered ischemic. I think we have seen enough evidence that ischemia transiently damages the heart and I am against damaging the heart. So, I would do something to prevent him from having ischemia.

Dr. Gibson: I also would do a thallium test. There are really two issues here. I think you have to view the exercise test in an apparently healthy asymptomatic individual relative to its diagnostic and perhaps more importantly its prognostic capabilities. We might ask what is the predictive value of painless ST segment depression in an asymptomatic individual for angiographic coronary disease and if you look at the 3 studies that have addressed that issue, and I believe those 3 studies include about 336 patients, only 86 or 21% of patients with definitely positive exercise tests had any angiographic coronary disease. The point being that most positive tests in an asymptomatic individual are false positives. So you really have to be very cautious in labeling the patient as having anything other than ST segment depression during exercise. Of course, once that is documented, it creates a problem. It potentially can lead to some psychological difficulties with the patient and of course can lead to some problems with insurability and of course has implications in those individuals engaged in hazardous occupations such as commercial or military aviation, policeman, fireman, etc. The other side is the prognostic value. Despite the inability of the exercise test to really give you information that is diagnostic of coronary disease, it does seem to indicate that an abnormal ST segment response increases the probability of some clinical manifestation of coronary disease in the future. If remembering the data that Dr. Selwyn presented, there are 3 other studies on top of the 4 he presented and if one pools all of the data from those 7 studies in over 16,000 patients, the risk of an asymptomatic patient who shows an abnormal ST segment response to exercise of having an event relative to his counterpart with a normal ST segment response, is 4.2 to 1. Most of the events seem to be angina. There is one study, a study by McHenry which demonstrated that an abnormal ST segment response while predictive of angina is not associated with an increased risk of mortality or myocardial infarction. I think we should not lose site of that study, that needs to be pursued. Certainly it should be emphasized. What would I do? I would probably go to coronary arteriography directly if the patient demonstrated ST segment depression at a very low work load or if the ST segment depression at a low work load and heart rate was associated with exertional hypotension. I would not rely entirely on the ST segment response. I would look at other variables, such as the blood pressure response, the time to onset, the amount of ST segment depression etc. If it was associated with hypotension in the first stage of Bruce protocol it is associated clearly with an increased risk and I think in those patients we need not do another non-invasive study and just pursue coronary arteriography. What about the patients? The more typical patient is one who shows ST depression at high work loads. In that patient I would perform stress perfusion imaging because studies have demonstrated that there is important additional diagnostic and prognostic information. The largest study was a study published by Euell in 1981, where he looked at 195 asymptomatic patients all of whom had ST segment depression, coronary arteriography, and thallium scintigraphy. There were only 21% of the patients in the entire group with coronary disease, but they demonstrated that a normal thallium scan in a patient with a positive stress test reduces the probability of coronary disease from 22% to less than 1%. So a negative thallium scan is helpful. A positive thallium scan in that population improves the probability of finding important coronary disease to 74%, finally the study that was published in abstract form from Baltimore, demonstrates that if you stratify patients with abnormal ST segment responses based on the presence or absence of the thallium abnormality you do identify better the group that truly is at risk of major cardiovascular morbidity and mortality. That was published in 1984. It was only 34 patients, all of whom had abnormal ST segment responses. Twenty had normal thalliums, 14 had abnormal thalliums, but the cardiac event rate in the latter group, the abnormal thallium group was 38% versus only 4% in the normal thallium group and that represents a risk ratio of 7.1.

Dr. Morganroth: It sounds like you would get a thallium.

Dr. Gibson: I would get a thallium.

Dr. Morganroth: What if the thallium was abnormal. Would you treat the patient with medicines or would you go on to coronary angiography.

Dr. Gibson: If the thallium was normal, I would do nothing. If it is abnormal, my decision would be based on the amount of ischemia. If there was an extensive amount of ischemia, particularly ischemia involving the territory of the LAD I would pursue coronary arteriography. If it was a small amount of ischemia, I would first intensively attempt to modify risk factors and secondly place the patient on prophylactic medical therapy.

Dr. Morganroth: So it sounds like you have a similar answer to Dr. Cohn, you don't seem to disagree with each other.

Dr. Selwyn: I would be guided by the time at which the ST segment depression came on and the strength of the ST segment depression. I think it should not be used to try and predict coronary disease at all. It should be used only as an indicator of risk and as such, once the ST depression is 2 mm or more, the problems of sensitivity and specificity are irrelevant for individual patients because it is sufficiently high to mark that patient as having a 5 to 15 times increased chance of coronary events on follow-up. So the implications for that patient over the next 10 or more years are very important if they have coronary disease or if they do not and if the test was intermediate obviously positive or strongly positive, I would recommend coronary arteriography because it is the only investigation that follows that has an order of magnitude of predictive and prognostic power enough to guide your hand in future therapy.

Dr. Morganroth: So your answer is you would probably skip the thallium and go right to coronary arteriography to find out what you are dealing with specifically.

Dr. Selwyn: Unless as Dr. Cohn very wisely said, the man has a long exercise time and minor degrees of ST segment depression. There I agree with him entirely.

Dr. Morganroth: Do you treat asymptomatic moderate coronary artery disease?

Dr. Selwyn: It is difficult to understand what moderate coronary artery disease is, but if the man does not have severe proximal three vessel disease, a damaged left ventricle or left main stem disease but has an obviously positive exercise test, with important stenosis of epicardial arteries, yes, I would undoubtedly treat him by risk factor reduction, I would try to reduce or control the ischemia. If it was a technically low risk and obviously positive exercise test, many of the groups in this country would try angioplasty as well.

Dr. Pepine: I would use the same criteria that were mentioned to try to risk stratify the patient based on the exercise response. I would add to a worrisome test the criteria of the onset of ischemia at a low work load either 6.5 METS or lower or a heart rate of 120 or lower. Also add to it the presence of ST segment shifts in multiple leads that reflect multiple surfaces of the heart and ST segment depression that persists for a very long time usually the cut-off is about 6 minutes into recovery. Also, ST segment depression that is associated with a fall in blood pressure should be added. I think there are a number of studies that show that those are factors that predict very high risk of events and then if the patient has those findings. I would move to an anatomic study to see if I could identify anatomy that is associated with high risk and if I did, I don't think that it would be a problem in my way of thinking to operate or pursue angioplasty if I identified anatomic features associated with high risk.

Dr. Gottlieb: First, my opinion is the same as the rest of the panel but I think our practice perhaps exceeds our knowledge in this area. We really have no results of any randomized trials showing that specifically treating asymptomatic ischemia in any way lowers the risk for future events and this is something we need to see.

Dr. Morganroth: It appears that our faculty have a unanimous opinion that they would pursue a diagnostic test in someone who they suspected might have underlying coronary disease which has manifested itself only as asymptomatic electrocardiographic ST changes. There was a slight difference in the treatment aggressiveness where some would favor a medical approach where others would favor even a surgical approach in totally asymptomatic patients if their anatomy was frightening to the eye. Let me ask Bob Temple to complete this question by giving his thoughts about what he has just heard, particularly is silent ischemia a real entity?

Dr. Temple: One couldn't argue that there isn't such a thing as silent ischemia and the overwhelming epidemiologic evidence it seems to me shows that it has something to do with prognosis, that it is a risk factor. But seeing that doesn't really tell you much about what to do as far as treatment because the fact that something is a risk factor does not tell you anything about mechanism directly. It may be an index of something else. It may tell you about the significance of anatomy or the significance of collateral circulation or any one of a number of things. Just to cite examples we all know about, we all know that post-infarction patients die suddenly of presumably of arrhythmias, but it is still an open question of whether treating such patients with antiarrhythmics (which is a perfectly logical thing to do given the mode of exodus), improves the prognosis. In addition we know that having arrhythmias of a certain degree on the electrocardiogram after infarction is a risk factor, so the situation seems to me very similar in that we know something is a risk factor, we have a logical way of dealing with it, but it isn't self evident to dealing with it in that way improves anything. The comments about treatment said a number of things. The first and sort of obvious thing is that if you know that a person has one more risk factor, you might try to treat all the others. You might try to get them to lose weight, stop smoking, calm down, things like that. Conceivably you would be more aggressive about cholesterol at the margin, but it still seems to me that there is an important question to ask about how you would treat this. Let me just make one or two more points. In the post-infarction setting, which doesn't seem entirely dissimilar, we are talking about people with similar kinds of anatomical problems and similar kinds of death. It is pretty clear that certain members of a class of drugs have a favorable effect on survival through mechanisms that are uncertain. That class of drugs happens to be anti-anginal but it isn't clear that the anti-anginal effect of the drug is what is good about it. Other classes of anti-anginal drugs, at least thus far have not been studied well enough perhaps but have been studied some, have really not been shown to have a favorable effect on survival. What is the implication of that? If one is trying to treat the risk factor and reduce the threat of death or infarction, what does that imply about which drug to use. Is it logical to say that any anti-anginal drug or any anti-ischemic drug is equally likely to make sense or beta blockers and calcium antagonists and nitrates all in the same bag here? You have one kind of evidence in the post-infarction setting with one of those classes and no evidence on the other. Again, that all goes to whether what we are talking about here is a mechanism or an indicator and I think it is hard to argue that there isn't an indicator and I wouldn't do that, but it doesn't obviously imply something about mechanism. I am struck by the fact that when people talk about the post-infarction studies with beta-blockers, there is a lot of talk about how it changes your lifestyle to go on a beta blocker and you should only pick the people who are at highest risk and yet there we have actual studies, hard numbers that show that you improve survival and to some extent even in the low risk patients. Here there isn't really any evidence at all that you will enhance survival, and yet there is some thought that these people ought to be treated or at least a lot of them ought to be treated. There seems to me at least some possible inconsistency there. On the other hand faced with a patient with horrible ST abnormalities at an early stage of exercise, I am not sure that anybody could resist trying to do something.

Dr. Morganroth: Ray, do you have anything to add to that?

Dr. Lipicky: No I really don't.

Dr. Morganroth: Anyone on the panel have anything to add to what Dr. Temple just said.

Dr. Selwyn: If you deal with managing patients rather than regulatory issues, the first order of business is to relieve symptoms, and the second order of business is a genuine attempt to shift people from high risk groups to low risk groups. It is only a third order of business when available to follow the dictates of clinical trials.

Dr. Temple: How do you know when you are doing that? Are you making an educated guess, which is probably a reasonable thing to do.

Dr. Selwyn: There is no guessing the first dictum of relieving symptoms. There is no guess, it is either practiced or it isn't. The second guess is that if you look at people who do have ischemia or a lot of ischemia, they are at high risk. Do you leave it or do you try to shift them to a low risk group, in other words, an individual who doesn't have any ischemia. That is a rational attempt that he is now in practice because physicians vote with their feet on the thought that they would rather their patient be in the low risk category than in the high risk. What follows is a necessary third step and that is controlled trials which you have not yet done to prove that that in fact can be done, but because of the frailties of these kinds of trials, one cannot simply wait and this is particularly in extreme cases for these trials to be completed, finished, approved and then reconfirmed. It is not possible because of the frailty in the whole ideal of doing clinical trials in this way.

Dr. Morganroth: How do you know when you go from an alleged high risk group by eliminating that risk factor that you are now in a low risk group? That is a leap of faith.

Dr. Selwyn: You look at both sides of the coin and the observational studies that have been done. One side of the coin is that if patients groups or individuals do have ischemia, they have increased risk, then you turn and look at the other side of the coin, what about similar patients who don't have ischemia, they belong to low risk groups. So it is a rational but not proven notion that it is a good thing to shift your patient from a high risk group to a low risk group, but I admit with you it is a rational notion but not a proven notion. The third category is a frail one. That is you have to perform these clinical trials and wait to overcome the frailties and prove your point. I don't leave it out, but I do place it third.

Dr. Temple: I am still curious about the choice of therapy. I mean in the post-infarction setting where I presume the same kinds of things are going one, although one doesn't always know, there is rather solid evidence that certain beta blockers have a favorable effect on survival and there is really no evidence that anything else does. Does that imply using the same kind of analogy and reasonableness criteria that you are suggesting is the only choice when there is no clinical trial data, that one should emphasis the class that is known to have a favorable effect, or doesn't it matter.

Dr Selwyn: Once you get into choosing therapy or clinical therapeutics, you have a number of issues quite apart from the one that you have raised. The first one is that the side effects of the agent have to be, or the risks of giving the agent, have to be considerably less than the risks that you have estimated for the patient's condition and that guides your hand as much as any of the other issues that you have chosen. It is true that if you look for the choice of an agent, you would ask it to shift the patient from high risk to low risk by observing the individual. Your hand might be guided when such clinical trials have been done, certain beta blockers after infarction, you have fulfilled the third set in the three that I described and that is useful information. I grant that it should be used. Many of the other drugs have not been tested and so there is a lack of information rather than saying that they do not produce the same effect.

Dr. Gottlieb: I think in terms of the post-infarction therapy issue, if the beta blocker studies were stopped at a level of which a number of other anti-ischemic drugs have now been studied, we might still be concluding that the beta blockers also are not useful. In my mind, the two analogies that one has to choose from in terms of dealing with the patient in front of you now, is it like PVC's that are occurring in asymptomatic individuals in which a number of studies, show that in the absence of other significant evidence of heart disease they have little prognostic significance. Or, is it more like hypertension, an asymptomatic condition that produces a very high risk of subsequent events? It is my personal opinion that silent ischemia is more like hypertension than PVC's.

Dr. Cohn: The example of hypertension is an excellent one. Many years ago before the various hypertension trials were completed, physicians who treated high blood pressure did so without any firm foundation as clinical trials but intuition of the physician that a blood pressure of 200/150 somehow was not what God intended you to walk around with and bad things would happen. Clinical trials subsequently verified that. Dr. Temple sounds very much like house officers at my institution. Unless I can show them a p value of at least less than .05 in the New England Journal of Medicine they refuse to do anything. Their attitude is it hasn't been proven yet. A physician is more than just a scientist. He must deal with people who have problems. He must use his observational sense and he must know when something is on the cutting edge and when something isn't. There have been several studies we are all familiar with which did not achieve that statistical significance when they first appeared, and years later when more patients accumulated etc, all of a sudden it became proper to do something in 1986 that it wasn't proper to do in 1983. I am not even referring to silent ischemia at all. The physician has to be guided by some sense of observational power and intuition as long as he follows the rule that Dr. Selwyn mentioned. As long as he doesn't do any harm to the patient, and that is the key thing. I don't personally think it is good for the heart to be constantly ischemic and you have seen evidence to that. If I can give a patient medication to prevent this and not cause undesirable side effects, I will do so.

Dr. Pepine: I would like to take up where some of my colleagues have started and maybe provoke the FDA a little bit. I would assert that part of the problem we are having with this discussion relates to the fact that the FDA continues to maintain an anti-anginal indication rather than an anti-ischemic indication. In the discussion that we have had so far, I didn't see Bob Temple flinch when he talked about antiarrhythmic therapy yet there are virtually no data that treatment of these PVC's that he mentioned had anything to do with prognosis yet he refers to it as antiarrhythmic therapy rather than anti-palpitation therapy which is not a recognized indication. The same was mentioned relative to anti-hypertensive therapy, and there are virtually little data in the mildly hypertensive individual that we do very much and when the data did arrive, what little data that we have, it just came and I remind you that Roosevelt died from untreated hypertension at least not vigorously treated hypertension and a lot of other people have died from the same thing because people did not have data. We did the same thing really with the cholesterol data, the guidelines that were just announced with an LDL of greater than 160, we have little data that will alter risk in that subset group of patients, yet we accept that, but in ischemic heart disease we are tied into this ischemic heart disease equals pain, pain means angina, anti-anginal agents are to be given to relieve symptoms. We have lost touch with the idea that pain is really a minimal part of the syndrome, the basic pathophysiologic problem is ischemia and unless we get into treating ischemia I don't think we will ever be able to make that break until 10 to 15 years from now as Andrew mentioned when we have hard data relative to survival and then we will come back and say, gee we should have looked at that 10 years ago. Look at the patients we might have saved. We have good evidence in the very severely ischemic individuals which is those who have left main disease regardless of whether they are asymptomatic or not to show that relieving ischemia prolongs survival. It seems to me that it is just as logical to extrapolate that as a high cholesterol down to the mildly ischemic individuals or to the high degree of blood pressure elevation down to the mildly hypertensive, but yet we reach this barrier that with no pain the patient is fine.

Dr. Lipicky: It seems to me that it is a misconception that you have. The drugs that have FDA approval have two characteristics. One is that they relieve anginal pain and the second is that they are anti-ischemic. The requirement for approval is that a drug have both properties. You are perfectly capable in the absence of an FDA statement of some sort or another to use exactly the rational you were. I don't see how you can lay that at the feet of FDA.

Dr. Pepine: Having reviewed your guidelines recently, I fail to see that statement. As a matter of fact as I recall the guidelines...

Dr. Lipicky: Which guidelines did you read?

Dr. Pepine: The last issue that you have. It is a mimeograph sheet that you circulate to industry.

Dr. Temple: He is trying to get you to say they are anti-anginal guidelines.

Dr. Lipicky: If you read them it says that an anti-anginal drug must both affect pain and have anti-ischemic components.

Dr. Pepine: I quess we are discussing apples and oranges. What I am saying is that if you focused on ischemia, pain would go away if it was related to ischemia. If you focus on pain, you have no idea what ischemia is doing. Your guidelines focus on pain.

Dr. Lipicky: No, they focus on both.

Dr. Pepine: Then I am reading something different.

Dr. Lipicky: It may be poorly written, but the intent of the guidelines is that one must demonstrate both components in that an anti-pain component in the absence of the clear demonstration of an anti-ischemic component would be inadequate and vice versa. That is demonstration of a clear anti-ischemic component without a demonstration of an anti-anginal component would be inadequate also. Dr. Temple: It is possible that someone ought to try to write an anti-ischemic drug guideline. That is sort of what these two days are about. Let me make one observation. I think it is fine to say that the third phase of knowing things is clinical trials to demonstrate it and that physicians have to take actions before they know that. You can't sit there in the face of patients and necessarily wait for all the evidence to be in and that you rely on "observation and intuition". I guess my observation would be that what we are talking about here is intuition and I don't understand what observation has to do with it. You can't by observing individual patients reach the conclusion that the prognosis is improved by treating what is a risk factor. That kind of data can't lead to that conclusion. Intuition is a fine basis for doing things, you have to use that, and one can't argue with it. What troubles me I think that what is based on intuition and what is based on hope and logic, fairly quickly becomes perceived as the standard and necessary treatment. That is what I really hear in what Carl Pepine is saying, that plainly the boat has been missed here by failing to write labeling that says "Treat ischemia" that makes it rather difficult to even do the kinds of studies you are talking about and it seems to me that it blurs the distinction between what you have to do before you know quite what to do and what it is important to find out. To ignore for example the fact that only one class of agents has been shown to be effective in the post-infarction setting and say that that doesn't matter very much, it seems to me undercuts the whole idea of trying to improve the prognosis. We don't know enough, and finding out is very hard because it takes huge trials and a long time and this is not an easy situation by any means, but there are only a few linch pins. Sometimes things don't work out the way you expect them to, for example, while hypertension is plainly associated with coronary artery disease, it has been difficult or impossible depending on who you believe to show the treatment of hypertension helps that. It helps heart failure and it helps stroke, but what its impact or what the drugs studied do in coronary artery disease is not so clear and that may be because the drugs had other things that went the other way, so even that is not so clear. Finally, I want to say on antiarrhythmics, we are trying to correct what we perceive to have been in error and now most of the new labeling for the new agents says "For the treatment of symptomatic arrhythmias" and it says we don't know if it is useful to treat asymptomatic arrhythmias. That doesn't mean that physicians won't choose to do it, and we don't care if they do, but as far as the evidence that it is useful goes, we don't think there is any. I think most of the people would have to say that is true.

Dr. Cohn: Let me make a point please about observational material. What I meant to say by that was observational in the sense when we know that prognostic studies implicate silent ischemia as an adverse prognostic sign, that's observational. Secondly, I have to take extreme objection to you keep referring to ischemia as only a risk factor, like we are going to correct cigarette smoking so that is a risk factor and ischemia is a risk factor. It is very different. Ischemia per se damages the heart. Every time there is an ischemic episode, there is some damage to the function or metabolism of the left ventricle. This has been well demonstrated. It is more than just an academic argument about some future risk factor, it is actually happening at the time to the heart.

Dr. Selwyn: I would take issue with the word intuition. I think that it is journalistic, inaccurate and inappropriate, because if you look at the background of knowledge and research that has been done, to show that the fundamental problem for these people is obstructive coronary disease, that its functional expression which damages the heart is acute transient ischemia and that acute transient ischemia can be entered into carefully controlled prospective parallel studies analyzed by multivaried analysis to be shown to separately be implicated in the adverse outcomes to these individuals. That those who don't have it do best and that those who do have it do worse. I therefore believe that when the clinical trials have been done which prove that the treatment of ischemia improves prognosis, that it will not be a great leap and new information that the lights will be turned on and everyone will understand, and in fact people will probably yawn and say "good lord, the background of information has been there, I am glad we have all been good boys and done the trials." It isn't intuition. I believe that there are at least 30 years of basic work applied physiological research and clinical research that has been done carefully and in good faith which supports these rational notions and the reason why physicians try to move their patients from high risk groups into low risk groups, it is not intuition at all.

Dr. Lipicky: I guess I am not sure what the discussion is about. I don't think anybody implied that any of the rationality that was being applied in the treatment in patients using the tools available was inappropriate or wrong and I don't think that anyone can say that from the vantage point of the requirements for approval of the tools that the standards that are being applied are wrong. I mean there certainly are anti-ischemic agents that are being made available. They also are anti-anginal. What are we arguing about?

Dr. Pepine: Here is what we are arguing about. The case that was presented that Joel Morganroth very carefully chose and illustrated a magnificent point led us down a pathway where a patient was totally asymptomatic and had the pathophysiologic manifestation of coronary heart disease and ischemia and Bob Temple mentioned that he would disagree with treating that individual because he wasn't sure what he was treating.

Dr. Temple: No I didn't. I think you should know the difference between why..

Dr. Pepine: Let's say it was my perception that a lot of physicians don't treat that individual because they are not quite sure what they are treating because their views are distorted because there is no classification in the current FDA approval system to treat such an individual because he doesn't have pain.

Dr. Lipicky: You mean medical schools and medical societies don't do anything? Just FDA tells physicians what to do.

Dr. Pepine: Let's just say that a practicing physician doesn't have an anti-ischemic drug or an anti-ischemic reason to think about ischemia when he talks about this particular patient so therefore this patient goes unmanaged in our view, because he can't make the barrier between here is ischemia and I have a packet of effective drugs and safe drugs by the way, much safer than the antiarrhythmic market, yet we have that antiarrhythmic indication. That is what we are arguing about.

Dr. Lipicky: You are arguing that there should be an anti-anginal/anti-ischemic?

Dr. Pepine: The other way, anti-ischemic.

Dr. Lipicky: So you think that semantic thing is going to change the picture of how the nation gets its medical care. Is that what you are saying?

Dr. Pepine: I am saying that that semantic thing has the potential to impact upon the outcome of a very very large number of patients, much more so than continuing with the semantics of anti-angina.

Dr. Temple: I take it the implication is that you feel that there is enough data now to allow people to advocate the treatment of asymptomatic patients with evidence of ischemia on the grounds that it will improve their survival, right? What would the basis other than that, for using a drug with an array of side effects..

Dr. Pepine: Relief or prevention of ischemia.

Dr. Cohn: Relief of ischemia to prevent damage to the heart.

Dr. Temple: And damage is manifested how?

Dr. Selwyn: It would probably be better to say the treatment of ischemia in itself to shift the patient from high risk to low risk.

Dr. Temple: But you don't know that you do that.

Dr. Selwyn: The rational notion from the pieces of research that you have seen is that those with coronary disease that have ischemia are at high risk and those who have coronary disease and no ischemia have low risk and all you can do is explain that the attempt in therapy is to shift people from high risk to low risk and you can follow that if you like with a sentence that the clinical trials are yet to be done to show that that individual would have a better chance.

Dr. Temple: But that is a plain statement that you are shifting him from one risk category to another.

Dr. Selwyn; That is correct.

Dr. Cohn: I would prefer to stick to the original point. If you can show that the ischemic episode causes metabolic and functional derangements of the heart, which we can, there is no doubt about that, you have seen data today for long periods of time. That to me would be enough to say that this should be prevented. With hypertension, when blood pressure goes way up and has its effect why should that be allowed to continue. Years ago it was. This is the episode that Carl Pepine was referring to. It was accepted practice 30 years ago to let people walk around with those blood pressures. I think today our state of the art has progressed. We know the damage that hypertension does. If we knew that 30 years ago, we wouldn't have to wait for those clinical trials. We know ischemia is a damaging thing to the heart.

Dr. Temple: It was accepted practice 20 years ago, at least partly because people had a rational reason, a wrong reason it turns out, a rational reason for thinking that you needed that head of pressure to get blood to the organs and they were afraid that they would all fail. Now we disregard that but it was a popular idea 30 years ago and was maintained by very respectable people.

Dr. Cohn: Suppose we could have shown 40 years ago that a hypertensive episode was damaging the kidney right on the spot like we can now for an ischemic episode of the heart. Then there would be a rationale for treating that hypertension, even though the clinical trials have not been done showing an increased mortality, etc. That is the point I am trying to make.

Dr. Ribeiro: Since there is conflicting data in the literature regarding post-MI patients with ischemia with or without pain, I would like to hear from the panel what is the concensus that they have for a post-MI patient with ischemia would be better off with or without angina.

Dr. Cohn: I think right now the evidence would seem to indicate based on all its studies, it probably doesn't matter. There are some studies that indicate that you may be somewhat worse off if you have angina plus ischemia and there are some studies that indicate that you won't. Dr. Weiner is going to talk this afternoon about the CASS experience which indicates it doesn't matter whether you have it or you don't have it. There are some other studies that you are a little worse off if you have angina. There is also a study from South Carolina that was published recently indicating that you might be a little worse off if you are painless. I think in the final analysis it is going to be the same sort of thing. If you have ischemia, that is the key. You are better off not having ischemia, that really is the question.

Dr. Ribeiro: Anyone else on the panel want to comment on that.

Dr. Gibson: I would agree with Peter Cohn. Rather than make decisions based on the presence or absence of angina since we have the techniques to measure and quantify the amount of ischemia, it makes more sense since in my mind prognosis is more intimately related to the amount of myocardium at risk. Our decision making should be based on the amount of ischemia. In patients with no ischemia, they have an extremely good prognosis. In patients with large amounts of ischemia regardless of whether or not it is symptomatic or asymptomatic, they have a terrible prognosis and of course there are a lot of patients that fall between those two extremes. The decision as to whether to cath and revascularize I think should be based on the amount of ischemia.

Dr. Gottlieb: I would suggest that it is a mistake to contrast silent versus symptomatic ischemia. I think that if you can summarize virtually all of the data that has been presented this morning, it is fair to say that we believe that angina is a relatively insensitive marker for the activity of coronary disease in ischemia and for that reason it is obviously helpful when its present but less so if it is not. I think that is a relatively simple concept but it gets obscured when one contrasts symptomatic and silent.

Dr. Temple: There is something that is known, although it isn't based on this distinction. Patients in the post-infarction setting, whether they have arrhythmia or not, whether they have angina or not are improved by certain beta blockers. That seems more important than some of this other stuff. I guess what continues to strike me is that I realize that there are areas in which you don't have all the data that you want and you have to rely on logic and that is inevitable. There are some areas where things have been studied. Certain interventions in people with coronary artery disease and who have manifested infarction, seemed to improve prognosis whatever the ischemic state of the heart. I mean aspirin does and certain beta blockers do. I guess that strikes me as important. I guess if I were exercising logic I would take those facts and apply them to people who haven't had an infarction yet and think that might matter.

Dr. Gottlieb: I think that is part of the problem in the clinical interpretation of these clinical trials. If you really look hard at which subgroups improve with anti-ischemic therapy, with beta blocker therapy, they are the high risk subgroups more than the lower risk. Bob Gibson and others have shown that calcium blockers in non-Q wave infarction patients have a propensity for recurrent ischemia. We have done studies with calcium blockers looking at reduced death and reinfarction rates with post-infarction ischemia and if you take the broad spectrum of all comers and lump the high and the low risk together, you are going to have difficulty finding out what is the mechanism of benefit. I think if one looks critically at the post-infarction clinical trial literature one can come to the conclusion that these high risk patients are the ones in which if ischemia is not documented, it is because it might not have been looked for number one or number two, it just wasn't looked for.

Dr. Riebeiro: I would like to know in data you showed, if you just do a correlation between the ST depression and the prognostic value, (disregarding the Thallium data), what result you get? Second do you find in your data any correlation between the magnitude of the ST depression and the perfusion defect by thallium.

Dr. Gibson: In answer to the second question, no we did not find a correlation because many of the patients that had ST depression did not have ischemia. I think in a certain relatively small subset of post-infarction patients, particularly those who have had occlusion of a large right or circumflex coronary artery, the ST depression was unassociated with chest pain (false positive). It is not an accurate marker of ischemia. In terms of your first question. If I apply that question to the current data set which includes 241 patients, ST segment depression by itself is a predictor of total cardiac events, those being defined as death, recurrent infarction or unstable angina requiring revascularization. One misses few patients relying on the ST segment response to exercise when the end point is death. However, in our experience and I think the experience of most others, the electrocardiographic response to exercise is a very weak predictor of risk of recurrent myocardial infarction such that if one were to lump the two hard events, death and/or reinfarction, one would not find a correlation. If one looks at the exercise studies that have been done since 1978, that have reported data on the predictive value of ST segment depression for death, one finds that of the 18 that have data that can be analyzed, 5 demonstrated that the ST segment response was a significant predictor. The other 13 found it to be only a weak predictor. My concern is reinfarction. I think that is an important event.

Dr. Ribeiro: Dr. Pepine mentioned during his presentation that he thinks that silent ischemia is more associated with the supply part of the equation than the demand and he showed beautiful data showing that metoprolol works very well in silent ischemia. I would like to ask him what the mechanism is for metoprolol working in silent ischemia?

Dr. Pepine: It made us recognize that the supply side is much more important in addition to the demand side. I am not in any way implying that the silent ischemic episodes are all supply side mediated. I think what happens is our myocardial oxygen demand does this all day. It starts out low in the morning, it increases with the catechol surge in the morning but it does oscillate throughout the day. Coronary flow or oxygen delivery does the same thing all day. It is related to some factors that we understand and some that we don't. When those two cross, then we have our ischemic episodes that occur during the day. A lot of those happen to be silent as opposed to the pure demand side, when you take a patient to the exercise laboratory, exercise him on a treadmill, the vast majority of those episodes turn out to be painful. That was the point. I am not saying that it is all supply side. I assumed that everyone recognizes that the demand side has a lot to do with it. Now we are much more focusing on supply also.

Dr. Wiener: I would like to make some comments from our studies. The first is that patients in the CASS study, the most important exercise predictor of prognosis was actually the final exercise stage. Among patients even with greater than 2 mm of ST depression, the survival varied by 40% depending on whether patients could exercise in stage 1 or less or stage 3 or more. The final exercise stage is the more important predictor of prognosis at least in our studies in CASS. The second point I would like to make is picking up on the theme of risk stratification, again in studies I'll show among patients with so-called silent ischemia during exercise testing, the event free survival can vary from 90% to 34% depending upon other factors such as coronary anatomy and importantly left ventricular function. So if you want to direct or target patients for aggressive therapy and that might just be even medical therapy as I hear, I think risk stratification is a very important feature. The third point is probably illustrated by a patient that was just referred to me last week. This middle age man who had symptoms of mild angina and the referring physician was going to do an exercise test as is commonly done and found that the patient had 2 mm of ST depression at stage 1 of the Bruce protocol. Then on my recommendation was referred to cardiac catheterization, but also on my recommendation the patient was treated with vigorous medical therapy. When he got to our hospital we got him on our treadmill again and now he can go 9 minutes on the treadmill Bruce stage 3 and had no ST depression. The house staff came to me and asked was this person considered high risk on the basis of his first exercise test or low risk on the basis of a second exercise test. Now he is on therapy. I think that is the crux of the matter that perhaps Dr. Temple was referring to. I cannot give any randomized control studies on that subject, but I can relate some of the data that we have from the CASS experience. In our high risk classification system which we defined as at least 1 mm in stage 1 of exercise, the prognosis was much lower whether or not patients were on medication or not. We separated patients who were treated with beta blockers and nitrates from those who were not. The prognosis was severely depressed not withstanding the medication. On the other hand, when we looked at our subset of patients who we considered to be lower as those patients who had no ST depression and could exercise into stage 3 or not, that prognosis was extremely good, again, whether or not they were on medication, whether or not patients had treatment with beta blockers or no treatment with beta blockers. That of course is not a randomized study and we haven't stated that they have an altered prognosis by medicine, but at least that gives you some idea and some data.

Dr. Morganroth: Dr. Selwyn, do you want to comment about the variability to risk stratifying patients from your data base?

Dr. Selwyn: One of the technical issues that concerns the detection of ischemia is, the measurement and the uses of an objective parameter in assessing progress. At present of course, I think that most of the guidelines confine their comments to the exercise test and ambulatory monitoring of the electrocardiogram in selected patients with known coronary disease. Showing obvious episodes of ST depression is more suited in many ways to looking at the effects of interventions or progress over prolonged periods of time out in daily life. I would have though of course from my own enthusiasm that this should be to supplement and clarify the effective agents on chest pain and to substantiate that in clinical trials. When you follow any of these biological signals over 48 hours or more, naturally there is great variability and if you are going to identify important changes you must understand the variability in perfectly stable people who are doing well. It turns out like all aspects of changing disease states, the variability is not small, it is great and for practical purposes of the management of a single individual one would have to produce a 80% or greater reduction. When it comes to clinical trials dealing with 10,20, and 50 patients, continuous monitoring shows itself to be very practical and one can detect significant change beyond a stable group with 95% confidence at a reductions of 20 to 30% which tell me that it is a definable method that can be used and controlled. So my own feeling is that one can get at least a numerical handle on the data and separate people who remain stable or who have important improvement.

Dr. Temple: We actually did use data of that kind for some of the unstable angina claims. Of course exercise tolerance doesn't help you so that I don't think there is any problem in using it.

Dr. Lipicky: It is in the current version of the guidelines as an acceptable means of demonstrating drug effect for an anti-ischemic claim.

Dr. DiPalma: Any patient that doesn't have symptoms and is told he has evidence of heart disease, is going to have symptoms after that and you are going to have to treat the symptoms at least. Another thing that hasn't been mentioned as therapy is nutritional therapy. Obviously what you want to do is reverse the process of arteriosclerosis if you can and I don't know if that is possible yet, but certainly one would look into the person's diet and see if they were eating the wrong things and perhaps we might even consider anti-lipidemic therapy even though the cholesterol is normal or considered normal. Now the question I have is that one of you, mentioned that he would not consider mass screening for ischemic heart disease and my question is based upon that statement. Suppose we took 1000 men 50 years old, randomly selected in the United States who had no risk factors for heart disease. They weren't overweight, they didn't smoke and they weren't hypertensive. Do we have any data how many of these men with a stress test would show some evidence of ischemic heart disease?

Dr. Pepine: One piece of data that may help, I recently saw an abstract from Framingham that looked at 2700 middle age men in Framingham and a comparable number of females with exercise stress testing. Ten percent of the Framingham population sampled, which was in that age band of middle age males which I think they defined as 35-55, had a positive exercise test and 5% of the females had a positive exercise test. How that translates to false positives, I am not sure. We don't know what that information means in the absence of risk factors. That is what screening would yield, I think that most of us would feel uncomfortable to say that out of 2700 asymptomatic patients, 10% have silent coronary disease. Nobody thinks it is quite that high and that is why we caution you about to mass screening. It is just too high with the techniques that we currently have available. One possible help is the computer processing of the electrocardiogram and I remind you of the MRFIT study which used a digitized electrocardiogram which was then processed off line to look at the integral under the ST segment rather than the physicians interpretation of ST segments. The physicians were notoriously poor with their visual interpretation and only when computer processed did the data identify a very high risk group. I don't think we have the tools yet to mass screen. It is not to say that we won't have it, but we'll pick up so many people in the screen that it will be mind boggling to try to deal with those numbers in our current limited state.

Dr. Cohn: Also the economics of it have to be considered because we are a cost-benefit conscious society and to look for the 5% of the population in the middle age males that have this particular problem by screening the entire population, you are going to find the ratio a false positive test, a true positive test, anywhere from 2 to 3 to 1 and to go through the necessary steps to weed out these true positives is going to be very expensive in terms of further non-invasive testing or coronary angiography plus the morbidity of such a procedure. If you take a look at a high risk group however, and the MRFIT is one of them, the lipid research clinic is another one, then a number of positive tests jumps markedly and your chances of finding disease are much better. You can have 20-25% of your population wrong and the chances are that a good number of them will have disease. So it makes sense from a logical point of view as well as from a cost-benefit point of view not to mass screen. One could argue on the other hand that you are going to be missing people. You are going to miss someone for some reason who doesn't have a high risk profile and he is going to die and this is all true, but to justify looking for the individuals and subjecting them to invasive procedures who might have disease, I think it makes much more sense. When I send this patient to coronary arteriography to confirm my non-invasive results, I know based on things you have heard the other people saying that I am going to get a 90% chance I am going to find disease. If I didn't have that liability and I sent someone for a cath procedure with only a 10 or 15% chance and they had some unfortunate event in the cath lab I would not feel very good about it nor would they. I think you must be very careful in that regard.

Dr. Morganroth: Would you advise the physician community to do an exercise test or a Holter monitor looking for ischemia in the population of patients who had at least 1 or 2 of the cardinal 3 major risk factors for coronary disease?

Dr. Cohn: One risk factor alone is probably not sufficient but I think if they had a combination of 2 or more and I am including the conventional ones plus premature atherosclerosis in the family at age less than 55 or so, and I'm not talking about women because I think they have a special problem, but men between the ages of 35 and 60, yes. Now, what test to do? I think that the chances of having a positive Holter finding in the absence of a positive exercise test are virtually nil perhaps with the exception of a silent Prinzmetal type. So I think that the exercise test at the present stage is an excellent screening procedure. I think the exercise test per se as a screening test in the person with 2 or more risk factors 35-60 year old male is something that I find indicated.

Dr. Morganroth: Compare that to the Holter monitor in terms of relative usefulness.

Dr. Cohn: I think that the Holter monitor as a screen is less useful because if you have a negative exercise test, you are going to have a negative Holter. On the other hand if you are going to have a positive exercise test, you may also have a negative Holter. The Holter comes in most importantly as angio has indicated and others are starting to show.

Dr. Selwyn: I agree with that because there is a long development in medicine of the exercise test and all of its information is so well understood and to some extent, Holter monitoring is new. I think that its sensitivity is very close to the exercise test and of course it has all the same specificity problems, depending on how you use it. The exercise test is of course desirable for all the reasons that you have listed, but I would say that the logistics of using it and the need for a laboratory and M.D. present and to some extent the expense will tend to make ambulatory monitoring more desirable. Technically ambulatory monitoring can be and will be easier to use as an initial screening procedure. Having said that the work that has been done that shows that it can effectively identify the subgroups at increased risk must be confirmed to support the idea that it could be used largely because it is physically much easier to use.

Dr. Agner: I would like to elaborate a little more concerning the treatment of that young man we heard about before, suffering from asymptomatic ischemia. As far as I understood the panel suggestions varied from do nothing to almost an immediate operation. My point is that looking at the study just reported by Blankenhorn and colleagues you might expect a beneficial effect of an aggressive medical treatment of cholesterol even at levels below 200 mg percent. In about 25% of the patients he treated the coronary stenosis was reduced and I think 50% of the patients I think didn't progress over a 5 year period. That study was done using medications with very many side effects. I think that you have now in the U.S.A. medications lowering cholesterol that virtually without serious side effects and I think there might be a point not just giving dietary advice but also treating very aggressively.

Dr. Morganroth: I think the panel frankly agrees pretty much with what you said. Most of them would want to decrease risk factors no matter what else they did because even if they went on to do an immediate operation, risk factor modification in such individuals is quite critical to prevent recurrent atherosclerotic disease.

Dr. Tuval: My question is angina or silent ischemia meaning ischemia per se whether it occurs during exercise meaning an increased myocardial demand in man versus when its due to decreased supply, do they carry different prognostic information, should we take that separate or complementary?

Dr. Pepine: I don't think we have the answer to the question that you are asking, but we could extrapolate from the data that we have talked about that the higher the work load or the higher the index of myocardial oxygen demand at the time that the ischemia is detected, the better the prognosis and the lower the index of oxygen demand with ischemia is detected, the poorer the prognosis. Therefore, if a patient has 2 mm or 3 mm of ST segment depression at a heart rate of 80 while he is sitting in his room, that should carry a poor prognosis compared to the individual who achieves a heart rate of 180 before he gets 2 mm of ST segment depression. Does that answer your question?

Dr. Tuval: I don't think so. I agree with you that exercise time and the magnitude of ischemia are related to prognosis. The question is, what is the additional prognostic information of seeing 60 minutes of silent ischemia.

Dr. Pepine: The only data that we have relative to that is Sid Gottlieb's data and the data from Brahma Singh suggesting that in unstable angina patients if you have prolonged episodes of ischemia in the CCU, that that group is a subset that has the worse prognosis. I don't know whether we can extrapolate that to the stable angina population. It is a possibility.

Dr. Gottlieb: We certainly know when symptoms are occurring at rest that that carries worse prognostic implications than symptoms only with extreme levels of exercise and then we call the patient with pain at rest unstable. When we have prolonged apparently unprovoked episodes at rest of silent ischemia there is data emerging that this is worse from a prognostic standpoint. So I think that certainly the magnitude of the risk assessment that the silent ischemia variables carries is comparable or in the same direction as that that we see with angina.

Dr. Selwyn: Just to add some comments to your question for chronic stable angina outside of the hospital. Those of our patients who have positive exercise tests but who have no ischemia outside of the hospital occurring, particularly no ischemia with near the resting heart rate, have a very good prognosis even with a positive exercise test and in that group there are some positive at the end of stage 1 and in stage 2. In contrast as I showed you in those survival curves, those who have a positive exercise test, but in addition, have active ischemia out of hospital, belong to a subgroup with a significantly increased risk of adverse events, that may answer in part your question about the additional occurrence of ischemia at or near resting heart rates.

II. DETECTION AND PROGNOSIS

6

METHODS TO DETECT ISCHEMIA USING AMBULATORY (HOLTER) ELECTROCARDIOGRAPHY

HAROLD L. KENNEDY, M.D., M.P.H.

Division of Cardiology, Department of Internal Medicine, St. Louis University School of Medicine, 1325 South Grand Boulevard, St. Louis, Missouri 63104

Recent technical advances have led to important clinical progress regarding the understanding of the pathophysiology of myocardial ischemia and to its detection. Paramount among these advances had been the development of ambulatory (Holter) electrocardiography for the accurate electrocardiographic detection of the ST segment. Using this new technology, investigators have discovered that patients with varied forms of coronary artery disease have frequent episodes of ST depression both with and without symptoms. The lack of pain or symptoms has led to the clinical description of "silent myocardial ischemia". The veracity of this observation for indicating true myocardial ischemia has been attested to by validation studies using hemodynamic methods, radionuclide imaging, and angiography (1,2,3).

To understand the relative importance of ambulatory (Holter) electrocardiography and its use in detecting silent myocardial ischemia, it is important to understand the pathophysiologic sequence of myocardial ischemia and its events, methods that detect this sequential change, the electrocardiographic features which define ambulatory ECG silent ischemia, and to be knowledgeable about non-ischemic factors that affect the ECG ST segment and its interpretation. Moreover, a broad overview of studies using ambulatory electrocardiography monitoring in coronary artery disease and normal patients defines unique characteristics of ambulatory ECG ST segment changes observed in such populations (4). Studies to date have shown that ambulatory (Holter) electrocardiography has diagnostic, prognostic, and therapeutic assessment value in the study of silent myocardial ischemia.

Pathophysiology of Myocardial Ischemia

Myocardial ischemia occurs when myocardial oxygen supply does not equal myocardial oxygen demand. The most common cause is usually obstructive atherosclerotic plaque occurring in epicardial coronary arteries, but indeed may be due to any form of obstructive lesion. Experimental studies have shown and confirmed that when an epicardial coronary artery is occluded such as during coronary angioplasty, the earliest myocardial abnormalities are noted in diastole and are then followed by contraction abnormalities in systole (Figure 1). Such changes can be detected invasively by catheterization hemodynamic measurements (5) or noninvasively by echocardiography/Doppler (6). Subsequently, hemodynamic changes ensue with an elevation of left ventricular end diastolic pressure, followed by electrocardiographic changes (ST segment), and then the development of either angina or anginal equivalent symptoms. Noninvasive cardiovascular diagnostic tests which detect this sequence of abnormalities are depicted in Table 1. It has become increasingly recognized that the development of both electrocardiographic changes and symptoms of angina are a relative late finding in this sequence of ischemic intracardiac change.

Electrocardiographic Ischemia

Electrocardiographic ischemia can be detected by a standard 12-lead electrocardiogram, an exercise test, or ambulatory electrocardiography. The standard electrocardiogram utilizing 12 leads is the clinical mainstay diagnostic test to detect the ST-T changes of myocardial injury and ischemia. In clinical use, the standard electrocardiogram is used to assess persistent and current myocardial ischemia both with regards to its magnitutde (ST displacement) and extent (number of leads) (Table 2). The standard electrocardiogram is often used to assess transient complaints of chest pain which may represent transient ischemia, particularly as a diagnostic test for complaints of atypical angina.

Exercise testing in contrast most commonly is used to examine for potentially inducible myocardial ischemia. Indeed, evidence of persistent or current myocardial ischemia would preclude performing an exercise test. Therefore, it is utilized to discover and reveal

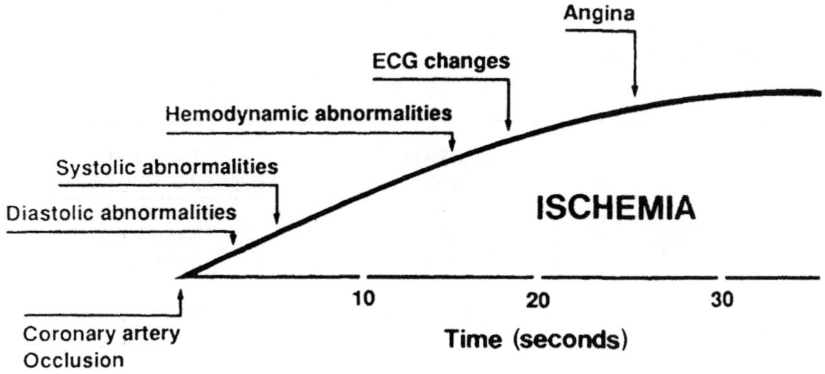

Figure 1. Pathophysiological sequence of developing myocardial ischemia . (Adapted from Siqwart (5).

Table 1. Cardiovascular diagnostic tests which detect the pathophysiologic sequence of myocardial ischemia.

Inadequate Perfusion →	Myocardial Perfusion (Thallium-201, Rubidium-82)
↓ Anaerobic Metabolism →	Positron Emission Tomography (C-11 Palmitate)
↓ Abnormal Wall Motion →	Ventriculography (Echo-Doppler, MUGA, Angiography)
↓ Abnormal Hemodynamics →	Systolic/Diastolic Pressures (Cardiac Catheterization)
↓ Electrophysiologic Changes →	Electrocardiography (ECG, Amb ECG, ExT)
↓ Chest Pain →	Clinical Assessment (Angina, Angina Equivalent)

MUGA = multiple gated acquition study; ECG = electrocardiogram; Amb ECG = ambulatory electrocardiogram; ExT = exercise testing

TABLE 2: Electrocardiographic differences of the standard electrocardiogram (ECG), exercise test (ExT), and ambulatory electrocardiogram (Amb ECG).

	ISCHEMIC TYPE	ISCHEMIC CHARACTERISTICS
ECG	Persistent Current	Magnitude Extent
ExT	Potentially inducible	Magnitude Extent
AMB ECG	Spontaneously occuring episodes	Frequency Duration

TABLE 3: Factors that affect the electrocardiographic ST segment

Ischemia
Myocardial infarction
Ventricular hypertrophy
Electrolyte imbalance
Conduction disturbance
Autonomic changes
Pharmacologic agents

potentially inducible myocardial ischemia. Similar to the standard ECG, exercise testing when utilized with a 12 lead electrocardiogram will also reveal the magnitude and extent of ischemia.

Ambulatory electrocardiography in contrast is used during normal daily activities to assess myocardial ischemia which occurs spontaneously and may or may not present symptoms. When utilized in this setting, ambulatory electrocardiography provides an assessment of both the frequency and duration of myocardial ischemia that occurs throughout a 24 hour diurnal cycle (Table 2).

In assessing myocardial ischemia with electrocardiographic detected ST segment changes, it must always be borne in mind that the electrocardiographic ST segment is affected not only by myocardial ischemia (angina or myocardial infarction), but also by ventricular hypertrophy, electrolyte imbalance, conduction disturbances, autonomic changes, and pharmacologic agents. These factors can affect every form of electrocardiographic detection, and must be taken into account before concluding that a detected ST segment change is due to myocardial ischemia. Additionally, other factors that affect the ambulatory ECG ST segment measurement include: 1) physiologic changes -- postural, temperature, post-prandial, autonomic, 2)signal characteristics -- frequency response, phase response, amplitude/noise relationship, and baseline stability, and 3)interpretive factors -- Computer and visual accuracy, episode criteria, and bipolar electrode lead positions. To decrease false positive factors involved in the accurate interpretation of the ambulatory ECG ST segment, workers in the field have defined the following criteria for ambulatory ECG silent ischemia, i.e., transient ST segment depression that is greater than 1 mm from baseline (without resting displacement) for 0.08 seconds after the J point lasting at least for 1 minute. Episodes have variously been defined as a return to baseline of this ST segment displacement for periods ranging from 1 to 3 minutes.

Ambulatory ECG ST segment abnormalities have been reported in normal subjects ranging from 0 to 39% (7,8,9,10). These false-positive studies in part resulted from a lack of clear morphologic interpretive criteria to define significant ambulatory ST segment changes, positional changes, bipolar leads used, and interpretive technical factors. In addition, Bayesian prediction of a higher false positive rate when such tests are applied to populations with a low prevelance of ischemic heart disease would be expected. Therefore currently, practical reliance on the ambulatory ECG ST segment as an indicator of myocardial ischemia should be confined to patients with documented coronary artery disease. Patients who have symptoms suggestive of coronary artery disease should most probably undergo some form of diagnostic testing that seeks the magnitude, extent and severity of ischemic heart disease. On the other hand, when such disease is detected, an assessment of spontaneously occurring ischemic events for both frequency and duration can be gauged with ambulatory electrocardiography. On a primary basis, ambulatory electrocadiography should not be used as the initial or solitary diagnostic test for coronary artery disease.

Characteristics of Ambulatory ECG Myocardial Ischemia

Numerous studies have now defined specific characteristics which are unique to the ambulatory ECG detection of myocardial ischemia. The assessment of these spontaneously occurring episodes throughout daily activities has provided new insights into the pathophysiology of myocardial ischemia. Several observations are notable. First, in coronary artery disease patients, silent myocardial ischemia commonly occurs during usual daily activities and may be detected during exercise as well as non-exercise periods (2,11). Daily activities such as cold provocation, mental or emotional stress, or cigarette smoking have been substantiated to be causes of myocardial ischemia in coronary artery disease patients (12,13,14). Moreover, ambulatory ECG changes of ST segment most commonly are without symptoms (silent) and are found with a prevalence varying from 75% to 90%. Secondly, dependent on the state of the coronary artery disease patients, i.e., stable angina, unstable angina, nocturnal angina, etc., the prevalence of silent myocardial ischemia is correlated with a more severe degree of coronary artery disease (15). Third, examination of heart rates during the occurrence of ambulatory ECG ST segment changes discloses that evidence of myocardial ischemia occurs at heart rates 10 to 20 beats per minute lower than the same ST segment changes exhibited during exercise testing (2). This observation has given genesis to the concept that spontaneously occurring myocardial ischemia throughout the day is mediated by mechanisms other than myocardial oxygen demand. The latter observation has focused attention on normal autonomic vascular tone as well as coronary vasospasm. Fourth, examination of the most frequent time of occurrence of ambulatory ECG ST segment changes has revealed a typical circadian distribution with the highest frequency of episodes occurring during the hours of 6 am to 12 noon (15,16). This circadian variation parallels other pathophysiologic processes which have been associated with myocardial ischemia. When taken in total perspective, the data suggests that the increase in catecholamine and cortisol secretion seen in the early morning is associated with the pathophysiology of myocardial ischemia. These latter trigger factors can be responsible for increasing heart rate and myocardial oxygen demand, increasing vascular tone, increased platelet aggregation, and decreased fibrinolytic activity. Thus on the basis of these new observations, it is not difficult to hypothesize how myocardial ischemia can sometimes be induced at normal or low heart rates in the absence of an apparent increase in metabolic demand. Such a hypothesis is consistent with the observation that there is an increased risk of myocardial infarction, sudden death and death in the early morning hours (17,18,19). Therefore, ambulatory electrocardiography is valuable diagnostically in characterizing the frequency and duration of these spontaneously occurring ischemic events throughout a diurnal cycle.

Prognostic Value

Early studies with ambulatory ECG in patients with stable angina pectoris or post-myocardial infarction have demonstrated a subset of patients with spontaneous ST segment changes who are at increased risk of an adverse cardiac event (20,21). Many of these early studies were retrospective, subject to criticism in regards to technical aspects, but nevertheless were crudely consistent in showing an assocation of spontaneously occurring silent ischemia with an adverse prognosis.

More recently, prospective studies performed in hospitalized unstable angina patients have unequivocally demonstrated the prognostic value of ambulatory ECG detected silent ischemia in identifying a subset of patients at increased risk of cardiac events both in the short-term and long-term follow up (22,23).

Additional studies are needed to fully clarify the complementary role that ambulatory ECG detected ST segment changes will add to other prognostic clinical indices associated with outcome of coronary artery disease patients.

Ambulatory ECG Assessment of Therapeutic Interventions in Myocardial Ischemia

Ambulatory electrocardiography has been utilized to evaluate a variety of therapies directed at patients with myocardial ischemia. Studies of nitrates, beta-blockade therapy, calcium antagonist, platelet inhibiting agents, streptokinase, and coronary artery bypass graft surgery have all been evaluated for efficacy using ambulatory electrocardiography (24,25,26,27). Such studies afford an assessment of the benefits of these therapies in alleviating the frequency and duration of spontaneously occurring ischemia throughout daily activity. Given the limitations that the early studies evolved when technology for measuring ST segment changes by ambulatory ECG were in their infancy, nevertheless, the majority of observations appear valid in spite of any technical or interpretive criticisms that might be suspected. It is to be anticipated that therapeutic evaluation of myocardial ischemia in the future will develop a more critical set of guidelines to allow standardization and comparative assessment between various therapeutic regimens.

Importantly, other considerations which can affect therapeutic assessment should now be considered. As demonstrated in ambulatory ECG studies of cardiac arrhythmia and heart rate, the principle of individual variability and how it effects the spontaneously occurring frequency and duration of episodes of silent ischemia must be defined. Criteria establishing an objective assessment of specific therapeutic interventions for efficacy beyond the defined limits of variability must be found, and criteria to identify "pro-ischemia effects" which might result from some therapeutic interventions (such as vasodilators) must be identified.

BIBLIOGRAPHY

1. Chierchia S, Lazzori M, Freedman B, Brunelli C, Maseri A: Impariment of myocardial perfusion and functin during painless myocardial ischemia. J Am Coll Cardiol 1983; 1:924-930.
2. Deanfield JE, Selwyn AP, Chierchia S, Maseri A, Ribeiro P, Krikler S, Morgan MM. Myocardial ischemia during daily life in patients with stable angina: its relationto symptoms and heart rate changes. Lancet 1983; 2:753-758.
3. Biagini A, Mazzei MG, Carpeggioni C, Testa R, Antonelli R, Michelassi C, L'Abbate A, Maseri A: Vasospastic ischemic mechanism of frequent asymptomatic transient ST-T changes during continuous electrocardiographic monitoring in selected unstable angina patients. Am Heart J 1982; 103:13-29.
4. Kennedy HL: Ambulatory (Holter) electrocardiography and myocardial ischemia. Ann Intern Med (in press).
5. Sigwart U, Grebic M, Payot M, Goy JJ, Essinger A, Fischer A: Ischemic events during coronary artery balloon obstruction, in Rutishauses W, Roskamn H (eds): Silent Myocardial Ischemia. Berlin, Springer - Verlag, 1984 pg 29.
6. Labovitz AJ, Lewen MK, Kern M, Vandormael M, Deligonal U, Kennedy HL: Evaluation of left ventricular systolic an diastolic dysfunction during transient myocardial ischemia produced by angioplasty. J Am Coll Cardiol 1987; 10:748-55.
7. Stern S, Tzivoni D, Stern Z: Diagnostic accuracy of ambulatory ECG monitoring is ischemic heart disease. Circulation 1975; 52:1045-1049.
8. Armstrong WF, Jordan JW, Morris SN, McHenry DP: Prevalence and magnitude of ST segment and T wave abnormalitieis in normal men during continuous ambulatory electrocardiography. Am J Cardiol 1982; 49:1638-1642.
9. Quyyumi AA, Wright C, Fox K: Ambulatory electrocardiographi ST segment changes in healthy volunteers. Br Heart J 1983; 50:460.
10. Deanfield JE, Ribeiro P, Oakley K, Krikler S, Selwyn AP: Analysis of ST-segment changes in normal subjects: Implications for ambulatory monitoring in angina pectoris. Am J Cardiol 1984; 54:1321-5.

11. Deanfield JE, Shea M, Ribiero P, de Landsheerce CM, Wilson RA, Horlock P, Selwyn AP: Transient ST segment depression as a marker of myocardial ischemia during daily life. Am J Cardiol 1984; 54:1195-1200.

12. Shea MJ, Deanfield JE, de Landsheere CM, Wilson RA, Kensett M, Selwyn AP. Asymptomatic myocardial ischemia following cold provocation.
Am Heart J 1987; 114:469-476.

13. Freeman LJ, Nixon PGF, Sallabonk P, Reaveley D: Psychological stress and silent myocardial ischemia. Am Heart J 1987; 114:477-482.

14. Deanfield JE, Shea MJ, Wilson RA, Horlock P, de Landsheere CM, Selwyn AP: Direct effects of smoking on the heart: Silent ischemic disturbances of coronary flow. Am J Cardiol 1986; 57:1005-1009.

15. Quyyumi AA, Mockus L, Wright C, Fox KM: Morphology of ambulatory ST segment changes in patients with varying severity of coronary artery disease: Investigation of the frequency of nocturnal ischemia and coronary spasm. Br Heart J 1985; 53:186-193.

16. Rocco MB, Barry J, Campbell S, Nabel E, Cook EF, Goldman L, Selwyn AP: Circadian variation of transient myocardial ischemia in patients with coronary artery disease. Circulation 1987; 75:394-400.

17. Muller JE, Ludmer PL, Willich SN, Tofler GH, Aylmer G, Klangos I, Stone PH: Circadian variation in the frequency of sudden cardiac death. Circulation 1987; 75:131-138.

18. Willich SN, Levy D, Rocco MB, Tofler GH, Stone PH, Muller JE: Circadian variation in the incidence of sudden cardiac death in the Framingham heart study population. Am J Cardiol 1987; 60-801-806.

19. Mitler MM, Hajdukovic RM, Shafor R, Hahn PM, Kripke DF: When people die. Cause of death versus time of death. Am J Med 1987; 82:266-274.

20. Stern S, Tzivoni D: Early detection of silent ischemic heart disease by 24 hour ECG monitoring of active subjects. Br Heart J 1974; 36:481-486.
21. Johnson SM, Mauritson DR, Winniford MD, Willerson JT, Firth BG, Cary JR, Hillis LD: Continuous electrocardiographic monitoring in patients with unstable angina pectoris: Identification of high-risk subgroup with severe coronary disease, variant angina, and/or impaired early prognosis. Am Heart J 1982; 103:4-12.
22. Gottlieb SO, Weisfeldt ML, Ouyang P, Mellits ED, Gerstenblith G: Silent ischemia as a market for early unfavorable outcomes in patients with unstable angina. N Engl J Med 1986; 314:1214-9.
23. Gottlieb SO, Weisfeldt ML, Ouyang P, Mellits ED, Gerstenblith G: Silent ischemia predicts infarction and death during 2 year follow-up of unstable angina. J Am Coll Cardiol 1987; 10:756-60.
24. Frishman WH, Teicher M: Antianginal drug therapy for silent myocardial ischemia. Am Heart J 1987; 114:140-147.
25. Cherchia S, DeCaterina R, Crea F, et al. Failure of thomboxane A_2 blockade to prevent attacks of vasospastic angina. Circulation 1982; 66:702-705.
26. Krucoff MW, Green CE, Satler LF, Miller FC, Pallas RS, Kent KM, Del Negro AA, Pearle DL, Fletcher RD, Rackley CE: Noninvasive detection of coronary artery patency using continuous ST-segment monitoring. Am J Cardiol 1986; 57:916-922.
27. Quyyumi AA, Wright CA, Mockus LJ, Yacoub M, Fox KM: Effects of myocardial revascularization in patients with effort angina and those with effort and nocturnal angina. Br Heart J 1985; 54-557-61.

20. Stern S, Tzivoni D: Early detection of silent ischemic heart disease by 24-hour electrocardiographic monitoring of active subjects. Br Heart J 1974; 36:481-486.

21. [illegible]

22. [illegible] is [illegible] ... [illegible] technique [illegible] ... [illegible] angiography ... [illegible]

[illegible] ... 1983; [illegible]

23. [illegible] ... [illegible] for early [illegible] in patients with [illegible] angina ... Br [illegible] Med J 1983; [illegible]

24. [illegible] ... [illegible] silent ischemia ... [illegible] during [illegible] ... [illegible] angina ... Am J Cardiol 1987; [illegible]

25. [illegible]

26. [illegible] ... [illegible] ... 1986; [illegible]

27. Quyyumi AA, Wright C, Mockus LJ, Fox KM: Effect of [illegible] ischemia in patients with effort angina and those with [illegible] and nocturnal angina. Br Heart J 1985; 53: [illegible]

7

THE PROGNOSTIC SIGNIFICANCE OF SILENT MYOCARDIAL ISCHEMIA DURING EXERCISE TESTING

DONALD A. WEINER, M.D.

Department of Cardiology, The University Hospital, Boston University Medical Center, 88 East Newton Street, Boston, Massachusetts 02118

INTRODUCTION

Transient myocardial ischemia may occur during exercise testing in some patients with coronary artery disease (CAD) despite the absence of chest pain. A 20 to 40% incidence of asymptomatic ischemic episodes has been reported to occur during exercise testing in postinfarction patients and in patients with angina pectoris (1).

The clinical significance of these episodes lies in their association with future coronary events. Different outcomes may occur in different patient groups.

In postinfarction patients, survival is related to the occurrence of ischemic ST-segment deviations during exercise testing rather than to the presence or absence of symptoms. In a review of five studies employing exercise testing early after a myocardial infarction, Weiner found that depression of the ST segment occurs in 30% of patients after an infarction and confers a 36% risk of a coronary event and a 16% probability of cardiac death within an 18-month follow-up period (2). For patients without ischemic ST-segment depression, the risk of recurrent coronary events and cardiac death was 16% and 4%, respectively.

Even among the totally asymptomatic patient, the relative risk of an individual with ischemic ST depression during exercise testing developing future coronary heart disease was 10-fold greater than that of an individual with a negative exercise test (3).

The majority of ischemic episodes in patients with angina and CAD are silent (4). There still is controversy as to whether these painless ischemic episodes are as important predictors of future coronary events as are episodes associated with angina. Thus, we undertook a study to assess the prognostic significance of silent ischemia that occurred during exercise testing in patients with CAD and compared the outcome of these patients with another group of patients who developed both angina and ischemic ST-segment depression during exercise testing. Data from the Coronary Artery Surgery Study (CASS) registry consisting of a large group of well-studied patients with a long-term follow-up was analyzed (5).

The study population consisted of 1,899 patients from the CASS registry. The 880 patients with catheterization proven CAD (at least a 70% luminal stenosis) were divided into two groups: Group 1 consisted of 424 patients who developed at least 1 mm of ischemic ST-segment depression during exercise testing without the occurence of anginal chest pain, while group 2 comprised 456 patients who had both angina and ischemic ST depression during exercise testing. One thousand nineteen patients without CAD were used as controls.

RESULTS

The clinical characteristics, severity of CAD, and left ventricular function were similar among group 1 and 2 patients.

Three different endpoints at 7 years were analyzed: survival, absence from non-fatal myocardial infarction, and absence from sudden cardiac death (Table 1).

Table 1. Seven-year outcomes in groups 1 and 2

Endpoints	Group 1 (n=424)	Group 2 (n=456)	Controls (n=1019)
Survival	76%	78%	95% *
Absence of myocardial infarction	80%	82%	98% *
Absence of sudden death	91%	93%	99% *

* $P<0.001$

The cumulative seven-year survival rate was similar in groups 1 (76%) and 2 (78%). The other endpoints, absence of non-fatal myocardial infarction and sudden death, occurred in 80 and 91%, respectively, of group 1 patients and 82 and 93%, respectively, of group 2 patients. By contrast, the rates of survival, absence of myocardial infarction and sudden death were significantly higher in the control group compared with either group 1 or 2.

Among patients in group 1, both the survival and the absence of myocardial infarction rates were related to the severity of CAD and the presence of left ventricular dysfunction. Seven-year survival rates were 86%, 73%, and 57%, respectively, among patients with 1-vessel, 2-vessel and 3-vessel CAD ($P < 0.001$). 55% of patients in group 1 with depressed left ventricular function did not suffer a subsequent myocardial infarction compared with 83% of group 1 patients with preserved left ventricular function ($P < 0.001$).

DISCUSSION

Silent myocardial ischemia during exercise testing occurred in 48% of patients in our study. This rate was similar to the 43% prevalence rate by Falcone et al. (6) in patients with CAD and the 58% prevalence rate by Theroux et al. (7) in patients soon after myocardial infarction.

The results of our study indicated that transient myocardial ischemia during exercise testing has an adverse effect on long-term cardiac mortality and morbidity. Both the rates of survival and of subsequent acute myocardial infarction were similar among patients with ischemia whether it was accompanied by angina or not.

This study also identified subsets of patients with silent ischemia who are at greatest risk for future coronary events. Both extensive CAD and left ventricular dysfunction were powerful predictors of outcome in these patients.

CONCLUSIONS

Ischemic ST-segment depression without associated angina occurs frequently during exercise testing in patients with CAD. This finding confirms other studies showing that the majority of transient ischemic episodes during ambulatory monitoring occurs without symptoms (4). Since the long-term outcome of patients with myocardial ischemia is similar whether or not the ischemia is accompanied by angina, it is appropriate to recommend therapy to abolish both symptomatic and asymptomatic ischemia. More aggressive therapy should be directed to the patients at highest risk, those with extensive CAD and left ventricular dysfunction.

REFERENCES

1. Cohn PF. Prognosis and treatment of asymptomatic coronary artery disease. J Am Coll Cardiol 1983; 1:959-964.

2. Weiner DA. Predischarge exercise testing after myocardial infarction: prognostic and therapeutic features. In Wenger NK, editor: Exercise and the heart. Cardiovascular Clinics Vol 15/12, Philadelphia, 1985, F.A. Davis and Co., pp 95-104.

3. Weiner DA. The diagnostic and prognostic significance of an asymptomatic positive exercise test. Circulation 1987; 75 (Supp II): 20-21.

4. Pepine CJ. Clinical aspects of silent myocardial ischemia in patients with angina and other forms of coronary heart disease. Am J Med 1986; 80 (Supp 4c): 25-34.

5. Weiner DA, Ryan TJ, McCabe CH, Luk S, Chaitman BR, Sheffield LT, Tristani F, Fisher LD. Significance of silent myocardial ischemia during exercise testing in patients with coronary artery disease. Am J Cardiol 1987; 59:725-729.

6. Falcone C, DeServi S, Poma E, Campana C, Scire A, Montemartini C, Specchia G. Clinical significance of exercise-induced silent myocardial ischemia in patients with coronary artery disease. J Am Coll Cardiol 1987; 9:295-299.

7. Theroux PM, Waters DD, Halphen C, Debaiseux JC, Mizgala HF. Prognostic value of exercise testing soon after myocardial infarction. N Engl J Med 1979; 301:341-345.

8

The Role of Radionuclide Techniques in the Evaluation of Patients with Silent Myocardial Ischemia

B. Pitt, M. J. Shea

Division of Cardiology, Department of Internal Medicine, University of Michigan Medical Center, Ann Arbor, MI

Silent myocardial ischemia has been increasingly recognized and shown to be of prognostic importance. While most emphasis in the evaluation of patients with silent ischemia has been on the use of ambulatory electrocardiographic monitoring there is also an important role for radionuclide techniques. Radionuclide techniques are of value in: 1) The detection of myocardial ischemia; 2) in investigating pathophysiologic mechanisms; 3) determining prognosis; 4) evaluating the effect of therapeutic interventions. This discussion will emphasize the role of radionuclide techniques in patients entering trials to determine the effect of therapeutic interventions in patients with silent myocardial ischemia.

Before discussing the role of radionuclide techniques in the evaluation of patients with silent myocardial ischemia or asymptomatic coronary artery disease a brief discussion concerning the potential and limitations of radionuclide techniques in the evaluation of patients with ischemic heart disease is in order.

Exercise thallium-201 myocardial imaging was first reported by Bailey et al (1) for the detection of myocardial ischemia. Thallium-201 is taken up by viable myocardial cells in proportion to blood flow through an active sodium-potassium ATPase transport mechanism (2). Areas of myocardial ischemia can be detected by the finding of a relative decrease in tracer uptake (3). Ischemia is differentiated from infarction by the finding that in ischemia there is a gradual redistribution of thallium-201 into the area of ischemia such that after several hours the initial defect in tracer uptake is less obvious and the image more homogeneous. In part, normal myocardial cells tend to lose thallium over time while the initially ischemic cells lose thallium at a slower rate and may continue to accumulate thallium until equilibrium is reached. Areas of infarction tend to have a persistent defect over time. Care should however be taken in interpreting a persistent defect on a three to six hour thallium-201 myocardial reperfusion image since this time period may not be sufficient to allow complete redistribution of thallium-201 into the ischemic region (4). Positron myocardial imaging with F-deoxyglucose has shown that some areas of apparently persistent thallium-201 defects, initially diagnosed as being infarcted on the basis of the three to six hour redistribution images, contain viable myocardial tissue. Reperfusion of these areas by coronary artery bypass graft surgery has been shown to result in an improvement in regional myocardial wall motion confirming the presence of viable myocardium (5).

Recently isonitriles bound to technetium-99m have been suggested as a substitute for thallium-201 (6). These isonitriles are taken up by the myocardium in proportion to blood flow through a mechanism that is not completely understood. In contrast to thallium-201 the isonitriles do not redistribute. This is a disadvantage in the evaluation of the patient with suspected myocardial ischemia, since a separate exercise and resting image are required to differentiate ischemia from infarction. On the other hand, the technetium isonitriles given during a period of transient myocardial ischemia can be imaged several hours later and the initial area of ischemia still be detected by a decrease in tracer uptake, even though the area is no longer ischemic.

Radionuclide ventriculography with technetium-99m (7) bound to human serum albumin or red blood cells can also be used to detect myocardial ischemia. A normal left ventricle will increase its left ventricular ejection fraction by at least 5%, absolute, from a resting value of 50-70% (8,9). Patients with significant obstructive coronary artery disease will tend to decrease their ejection fraction during exercise and/or develop an abnormality of regional myocardial wall motion. Exercise radionuclide ventriculography has a sensitivity of greater than 90% for detecting patients with significant coronary artery disease, similar to that for exercise thallium-201 myocardial imaging, but in contrast to thallium-201 myocardial imaging has a lower specificity, depending upon the population studied. The reasons for the relatively low specificity of exercise radionuclide ventriculography for the detection of patients with anatomic coronary artery disease is due to the fact that several processes aside from coronary artery disease may lead to a decrease in left ventricular ejection fraction, or at least a failure to increase left ventricular ejection fraction by 5% during exercise. For example, infiltrative diseases of the myocardium; previous myocarditis; left ventricular hypertrophy; and patients with transient increases in afterload during exercise may fail to increase their left ventricular ejection fraction during exercise.

The finding of a positive exercise thallium-201 myocardial image and/or exercise radionuclide ventriculogram is suggestive of myocardial ischemia and the presence of significant anatomic coronary artery disease. Recent studies have however challenged the utility of a positive radionuclide stress test for the diagnosis of coronary artery disease. For example, the Cedars Sinai Hospital group (10) in reviewing their experience with radionuclide ventriculography noted that in the 1970's when the test was first introduced that patients referred to the cardiac catheterization laboratory who were found to have a normal coronary arteriogram tended to increase their left ventricular ejection fraction by at least 5%, absolute, from rest to exercise and had no or only minimal abnormalities of regional myocardial wall motion. However, in the 1980's they found that a large percentage of patients who had normal coronary arteriograms failed to increase their left ventricular ejection fraction during exercise and/or had an abnormality of regional myocardial wall motion. This study, suggesting a change in referral patterns in patients being studied in the catheterization laboratory cast doubt upon the diagnostic utility of the exercise radionuclide ventriculogram for the detection of patients with significant coronary artery disease. Similarly, investigators from the Massachusetts General Hospital (11) reviewing their experience with exercise radionuclide ventriculography found only a moderate sensitivity and specificity when a decrease in left ventricular ejection fraction was used to define the presence of myocardial ischemia. When they attempted to evaluate other parameters such as increase in pulmonary blood volume and the ratio of end systolic volume to end systolic pressure they had an increase in sensitivity but the specificity remained relatively low. Similarly, Wieshammer et al in examining a consecutive series of 56 patients referred to the cardiac catheterization laboratory for suspected coronary artery disease, without a history of prior myocardial infarction, found only a poor correlation between the exercise radionuclide ventriculogram and the presence of significant anatomic coronary artery disease. They concluded that exercise radionuclide ventriculography had little diagnostic value and that in the evaluation of patients with suspected coronary artery disease that it was more effective to proceed directly to coronary arteriography (12). While it is attractive in this era of cost containment to eliminate unnecessary tests, the decision to eliminate radionuclide testing in the evaluation of patients with suspected ischemic heart disease and those with silent or asymptomatic myocardial ischemia seems premature and unwarranted. On the contrary, a closer look at the available evidence suggests that the radionuclide techniques have an important role.

In part, the findings by the Cedar Sinai group (10), the Massachusetts General Hospital group (11), and Weishamer's group (12) may reflect the fact that patients referred to the catheterization laboratory for suspected coronary artery disease who are subsequently found to have angiographically normal coronary arteries may in fact not be free of ischemic heart disease and that the coronary arteriogram may be a poor "gold standard" by which to evaluate the radionuclide techniques.

Studies by Kubler et al (13) pointed out the fact that some patients with chest pain suggestive of angina pectoris who are found to have angiographically normal coronary arteries have on further testing a functional defect with reduced coronary flow reserve. Using Argon gas wash out techniques to assess coronary blood flow they found that patients with angiographically normal coronary arteries without a history of chest pain suggestive of angina pectoris had an almost fourfold increase in coronary blood flow in response to coronary vasodilatation with intravenous dipyridamole. Patients with a history of chest pain suggestive of angina pectoris but angiographically normal coronary arteries had a decreased coronary flow reserve, suggesting a functional defect in coronary vasodilatation. A positive exercise thallium-201 myocardial image or positive exercise radionuclide ventriculogram in such a patient would not be falsely positive but in fact a better guide to the presence of a functional defect than the coronary arteriogram which reflects only the anatomic situation. A similar situation has been found by Cannon et al (14). They have shown that patients with angiographically normal coronary arteries without a history of chest pain suggestive of angina pectoris tend to have a normal response to exercise radionuclide ventriculography, i.e. they increase their left ventricular ejection fraction by at least 5%, absolute. In patients referred with chest pain suggestive of angina pectoris who are found to have angiographically normal coronary arteries they found that some of these patients had a decrease in coronary flow reserve in response to intravenous dipyridamole while others had a normal flow reserve. Those with a decreased flow reserve but angiographically normal coronary arteries tended to have an abnormal exercise radionuclide ventriculographic response in that they did not increase their left ventricular ejection fraction by 5%, absolute, whereas those with a normal coronary flow reserve showed a normal response to exercise radionuclide ventriculography, increasing their left ventricular ejection fraction by at least 5%, absolute. Similarly, LeGrand et al (15) using digital coronary angiography to estimate coronary flow reserve (16) found that patients with angiographically normal coronary arteries but a positive radionuclide ventriculogram, exercise thallium-201 stress test, or both tended to have a decreased flow reserve, suggesting a functional defect not reflected by the coronary arteriogram. These studies point out the fact that the coronary arteriogram may not be an adequate "gold standard" for the evaluation of radionuclide studies that detect functional rather than anatomic ischemic heart disease. The relatively low specificity of the radionuclide techniques in some previous studies may reflect the fact that anatomic rather than functional criteria were used to define ischemic heart disease. Similarly, the low sensitivity for detecting ischemic heart disease by radionuclide techniques in some studies may reflect the fact that anatomic criteria such as a greater than 50% coronary artery narrowing rather than functional criteria were used to define ischemic heart disease. For example, in one study by Bateman et al (17) patients with significant angiographic coronary artery disease referred for surgery underwent rest and exercise radionuclide ventriculography. Despite the presence of angiographically significant coronary artery disease some patients had a normal rest and exercise radionuclide ventriculogram, while others while normal at rest had an abnormal response to exercise. Those who were normal both at rest and during exercise had a mean translesional pressure gradient of 10±6 mmHg, while those with an abnormal exercise response had a mean gradient of 24 ± 11 mmHg. In another study Bateman et al (18) found that patients with a 50-90% coronary artery narrowing had a negative planar exercise thallium-201 stress test and negative exercise radionuclide ventriculogram. In these patients with angiographically significant coronary artery disease but a negative exercise radionuclide study the mean translesional gradient was 10 mmHg (4-18 mmHg). A translesional gradient of less than 20 mmHg is considered an excellent result after elective percutaneous transluminal coronary angioplasty and is associated with relief of symptoms of ischemia. Ganz et al (19) have pointed out that in patients with documented 50 to 90% coronary artery narrowing at angiography that there is a wide range of translesional pressure gradients (0 to 55 mmHg) and a poor correlation between the angiographic presence of disease and its functional importance. In contrast, in patients with severe coronary artery narrowing, greater than 90%, there was a translesional gradient of 35 to 65 mmHg, implying functional significance. This finding is supported by the study of Bateman et al (18) in which patients with greater than 90% coronary artery narrowing had a mean translesional pressure gradient of 31 mmHg (18-48 mmHg), a positive planar exercise thallium-201 stress test and/or exercise radionuclide ventriculogram.

In part the relatively poor correlation between the presence of angiographically significant coronary artery disease and functional measures of lesion significance such as the translesional pressure gradient, exercise thallium-201 myocardial imaging, and exercise radionuclide ventriculography reflects the difference between the presence of significant anatomic and functional coronary artery narrowing as alluded to above and in part to the fact that the interpretation of the coronary arteriogram has for the most part been subjective with a wide inter and intra-observer variability. In the early days of coronary arteriography it was recognized that there was a great subjectivity in the interpretation of the coronary arteriogram (20). With increasing experience and wider application of the technique it was felt that the problem of interpretation had been minimized. However, the coronary artery surgery study (CASS) (21) completed in the 1980's in which some of the most experienced centers in the United States and Canada took part again demonstrated the variability and subjectivity in interpretation of the coronary angiogram. Angiograms sent from one CASS center to another showed good agreement in interpretation of percent stenosis only at the extremes, of no lesion or 100 percent occlusion. There was wide variability with lesions in the mid range. The limitation of the coronary arteriogram in the evaluation of patients with coronary artery disease can also be seen from a study by Jones et al at Duke University (22). In this study patients with significant anatomic coronary artery disease underwent rest and exercise radionuclide ventriculography prior to coronary artery bypass graft surgery. In some patients there was an abnormal rest to exercise radionuclide ventriculographic response while in other there was a normal rest-exercise radionuclide ventriculogram, despite the presence of significant anatomic coronary artery disease. The patients undergoing coronary artery bypass graft surgery were compared to matched patients in the Duke data bank who did not undergo coronary artery bypass graft surgery. The patients with an abnormal rest to exercise radionuclide ventriculogram prior to coronary artery bypass graft surgery had significant relief of symptoms and improved survival over a three year follow up period compared to those who did not undergo bypass graft surgery. In contrast, the patients with a normal rest to exercise radionuclide ventriculogram prior to coronary artery bypass graft surgery did not have significant relief of symptoms or improved survival over the three year follow-up period compared to the matched patients who did not undergo coronary artery bypass graft surgery.

The view that the radionuclide studies have an important role in the evaluation of patients with suspected coronary artery disease and those with silent or asymptomatic myocardial ischemia is further supported by the role of the radionuclide techniques in determining prognosis. Several studies have pointed out that a negative exercise thallium-201 stress test and or normal rest-exercise radionuclide ventriculogram is indicative of an excellent prognosis, with approximately a 1% incidence of cardiac events/year, regardless of the coronary angiographic findings or electrocardiographic findings. For example, Panelia et al (23) in a consecutive series of 349 patients with chest pain who underwent exercise thallium-201 myocardial imaging found that patients with chest pain and a normal exercise thallium-201 stress test had an event rate of 1.1%/year for cardiac death and nonfatal myocardial infarction, which is comparable to that in patients with chest pain and angiographically normal coronary arteries. Habibi et al (24) carried out exercise electrocardiography and planar exercise thallium-201 myocardial imaging in 1,939 patients. Of interest were the 114 patients with a strongly positive exercise electrocardiogram (> 2 mm ST segment change) but a normal exercise thallium-201 stress test. Follow-up on 107 (94%) for a mean of 3.3±1.2 years showed an event rate of 0%/death, 0.9%/year for myocardial infarction, 0.6%/year for coronary artery bypass graft surgery, and 0.6%/year for PTCA. The total event rate was 2% a year. They concluded that patients with a strongly positive exercise electrocardiogram and a normal exercise thallium-201 stress test have a low cardiac event rate similar to that reported for patients with angiographically normal coronary arteries. Johnson et al (25) in a series of 908 patients who underwent coronary angiography and exercise radionuclide ventriculography for suspected coronary artery disease and were followed a mean of 4.6 years found that those patients who had an exercise left ventricular ejection fraction of>55% had a cardiac event rate of 2% and a cardiovascular death rate of 1%. Also of interest is the study of Kotler et al (26) in 209 consecutive patients with significant coronary artery disease by arteriography who underwent exercise thallium-201 myocardial imaging and were followed for a minimum of one year without coronary artery bypass graft surgery. Exercise thallium-201 myocardial imaging produced a 20-fold risk stratification compared to a two-fold stratification by angiography alone, suggesting that exercise thallium-201 is superior to coronary angiography for prognostication. Similar results have been found for rest-exercise radionuclide ventriculography in patients with angiographically documented coronary artery disease (27).

Evaluation of Asymptomatic Patients with Suspected Ischemic Heart Disease

Electrocardiographic ST segment depression or elevation on exercise stress testing of asymptomatic or symptomatic patients with suspected coronary artery disease is most commonly used to select patients for inclusion in therapeutic trials of silent ischemia. Electrocardiographic ST segment changes may however be falsely positive, especially in women, patients on digitalis, and in those with baseline electrocardiographic abnormalities. ST segment changes on ambulatory electrocardiographic monitoring may also be due to changes in body position or artifact. For inclusion in a trial of therapy for silent myocardial ischemia asymptomatic patients should have evidence of myocardial ischemia independent of the electrocardiogram.

Caralis et al in 1979 (28) in one of the first studies of exercise thallium-201 myocardial imaging in the evaluation of silent myocardial ischemia examined 15 asymptomatic patients with multiple risk factors for coronary artery disease and a positive electrocardiogram. Of the 15 asymptomatic individuals with a positive exercise electrocardiogram five had a normal exercise thallium-201 myocardial image and ten developed a new thallium-201 defect with exercise. Four of the five individuals with a normal exercise thallium-201 stress test had normal coronary arteriograms and one an abnormal arteriogram. The patient with an abnormal coronary arteriogram had severe left main stenosis and triple vessel disease and was not detected as being abnormal in this early study by thallium-201 myocardial imaging but would likely have been detected using more recent criteria for the interpretation of exercise thallium-201 myocardial imaging. Of the ten with an abnormal exercise thallium-201 myocardial image, nine had significant multivessel coronary artery disease while one had minimal irregularities of the left anterior descending coronary artery. This study showed that exercise thallium-201 myocardial imaging had a higher predictive value than exercise electrocardiography in detecting myocardial ischemia in asymptomatic individuals with coronary artery disease. Uhl et al (29) studied 191 asymptomatic United States Air Force crewman with an abnormal exercise electrocardiogram, of whom 135 had a normal coronary arteriogram; 15 subcritical ($<$ 50%) coronary artery narrowing; and 41 angiographically significant coronary artery disease. Quantitative exercise thallium-201 myocardial imaging resulted in only four false positive and two false negative tests compared to the coronary angiogram. Of the 15 patients with subcritical ($<$ 50%) coronary artery narrowing, ten had a positive and five a negative quantitative exercise thallium-201 test. Kiat et al (30) studied 174 patients with angiographically documented single vessel coronary artery disease by exercise electrocardiography and quantitative planar and tomographic exercise thallium-201 myocardial imaging. They found that the exercise electrocardiogram had a sensitivity of 54% in those with angina pectoris and 57% in those without angina whereas tomographic exercise thallium-201 myocardial imaging had a sensitivity of 82% in those with angina and 92% in those with silent myocardial ischemia. They concluded that quantitative exercise tomographic thallium-201 myocardial imaging was superior to exercise electrocardiography for the detection of single vessel coronary artery disease, regardless of symptoms.

Investigation of Pathophysiologic Mechanisms in Patients with Silent Myocardial Ischemia

The mechanism of silent myocardial ischemia remains uncertain. Radionuclide techniques have however been of importance in the investigation of this phenomenon. Deanfield et al (31) studied 16 patients with stable angina pectoris who underwent exercise testing and mental stress with rubidium-82 positron imaging. They found that mental arithmetic caused 12 of the 16 patients (75%) to have an abnormal rubidium-82 uptake, accompanied by ST segment depression in six and angina pectoris in four. After exercise all 16 of the patients had a positive rubidium-82 response suggestive of myocardial ischemia, in the same areas affected by the mental arithmetic. These changes in rubidium uptake were accompanied by ST segment depression in all 16 patients and angina pectoris in 15. These studies indicate that episodes of silent myocardial ischemia induced by mental stress may have a similar location and extent as ischemia induced during exercise. Other investigators (32) using tomographic exercise thallium-201 myocardial imaging have also found that patients with angiographically significant coronary disease and chest pain and those with silent myocardial ischemia have similar amounts of ischemic myocardium. Hakki et al (33) using rest and exercise radionuclide ventriculography to investigate 118 patients with angiographically documented coronary artery disease and a normal resting left ventricular ejection fraction found 28 (24%) developed angina pectoris during exercise while 90 (76%) did not. The patients with angina pectoris had a similar severity of angiographic coronary artery disease and rate pressure product during exercise compared to those without angina pectoris. The patients who developed angina pectoris did however have a greater increase in left ventricular end systolic volume and a greater decrease in left ventricular ejection fraction during exercise than those with silent myocardial ischemia. However, even among those patients with the most severe left ventricular dysfunction during exercise (> 10% decrease in left ventricular ejection fraction) only 40% had symptomatic myocardial ischemia. Deanfield et al (34) in another study using rubidium-82 positron myocardial imaging in 13 chronic smokers with stable angina pectoris found that exercise induced angina pectoris and a positive rubidium-82 response occurred in eight (61%) of the patients. After smoking a single cigarette six of the eight with a positive exercise test had ischemia detected by rubidium-82 myocardial imaging in the same segment of myocardium detected during exercise. However, the episodes of ischemia during smoking were mostly silent and occurred at a lower rate pressure product than those occurring during exercise, suggesting an important role for an alteration in vasomotor tone and regional myocardial blood flow in the pathophysiology of silent myocardial ischemia.

The Role of Radionuclide Techniques in Determining Prognosis in Patients with Silent or Asymptomatic Myocardial Ischemia

There are relatively few studies of prognosis in patients with silent myocardial ischemia. The potential of radionuclide techniques can however be seen from the study of Asey et al (35). They studied 55 patients with angiographically proven coronary artery disease who underwent exercise thallium-201 myocardial imaging. Twenty-seven had evidence of ischemia without angina and 28 developed angina pectoris during exercise. The patients were followed a mean of 30 months. Six of the 27 (22%) with silent myocardial ischemia had a myocardial infarction on follow-up, three of whom died vs. one of 28 (4%) with angina pectoris, none of whom died $p < .05$. They concluded that silent myocardial ischemia detected during exercise thallium-201 myocardial imaging predicted a subset of patients prone to subsequent myocardial infarction independent of the angiographic extent of coronary artery disease and resting left ventricular ejection fraction. Clearly, more studies are needed to define the prognosis of patients with silent myocardial ischemia. The true prognosis in patients with silent myocardial ischemia will however require convincing evidence of ischemia rather than the ST segment response on the electrocardiogram alone or the demonstration of "significant" angiographic coronary artery narrowing alone.

Evaluation of the Effect of Therapeutic Intervention in Patients with Silent Myocardial Ischemia using Radionuclide Techniques

While ambulatory electrocardiographic monitoring has been most frequently used to evaluate the effects of therapeutic interventions in patients with silent myocardial ischemia it is evident from the studies referred to above that the electrocardiographic demonstration of a "ischemic" response may not be adequate to define ischemia nor therefore to assess the effects of a therapeutic regimen on ischemia in asymptomatic individuals. In one study by Cohn et al (36) the effects of beta adrenergic blockade were studied in 11 patients with angiographically documented coronary artery disease and silent myocardial ischemia during exercise using rest and exercise radionuclide ventriculography. There were 18 areas of jeopardized myocardium detected prior to institution of beta adrenergic blocking therapy. Before beta adrenergic blockade regional myocardial ejection fraction decreased in 15 of the 18 segments during exercise. After beta adrenergic blockade a decrease occurred in only six of the 18 segments, ($p < .05$). This study demonstrated that beta adrenergic blocking agents can relieve myocardial ischemia in patients with angiographically documented coronary artery disease and silent myocardial ischemia.

In summary, these studies suggest that a negative exercise thallium-201 myocardial image or normal rest-exercise radionuclide ventriculogram should be grounds for excluding a patient from inclusion into a trial of therapy for silent myocardial ischemia, regardless of the presence of a "ischemic" ST segment response on exercise electrocardiograhy and regardless of whether or not there is angiographically documented significant (>50%) coronary artery narrowing. This statement is based upon the fact that a positive exercise electrocardiogram in an asymptomatic individual is often falsely positive in comparison to the coronary angiogram and that a negative exercise thallium-201 stress test or rest-exercise radionuclide ventriculogram is associated with an excellent prognosis despite the presence of significant anatomic coronary artery disease on angiography. Use of the exercise or ambulatory electrocardiogram alone as the criterion for selection of patients with silent "myocardial ischemia" in asymptomatic individuals is hazardous since many of these patients may not have true ischemia. Similarly, reliance upon the coronary angiogram alone may allow selection of patients who have significant anatomic disease but do not have functional disease, ischemia, or a poor prognosis. Therapeutic agents such as nitrates, beta adrenergic blocking agents, and calcium channel blocking agents which act to relieve myocardial ischemia should be tested in individuals with documented ischemia to achieve the greatest chance of showing effectiveness and in altering the prognosis of those with true "silent myocardial ischemia".

References

1. Bailey, I.K., Griffith, L.S.C., Rouleau, J., Strauss, H.W. and Pitt, B. Circulation 55:79-87, 1977.
2. Strauss, H.W., Harrison, K., Langan, J., Lebowitz, E. and Pitt, B. Circulation 51:641-645, 1975.
3. Strauss, H.W. and Pitt, B. Am. J. Cardiol. 38:739-746, 1976.
4. Kiat, H., Maddahi, J., de Yang, L., Van Train, K., Daley, N., Wong, C. and Berman, D. Circulation 76:IV-255, 1987.
5. Schelbert, H. Can. J. Cardiol. Supp A:121A, 1986.
6. Liu, P., Houle, S., Mills, L. and Dawood, F. Circulation 76:IV-860, 1987.
7. Strauss, H.W., Zaret, B.L., Hurley, P., Natarajan, T.K. and Pitt, B. Am. J. Cardiol. 28:575-580, 1971.
8. Borer, J.S., Bacharach, S.L., Green, M.V., et al. N. Engl. J. Med. 296:839, 1977.
9. Brady, T.J., Lo, K., Thrall, J.H., Walton, J.A., Brymer, J.F. and Pitt, B. Radiology 132:697-702, 1979.
10. Rozanski, A., Diamond, G.A., Berman, D., et al. N. Engl. J. Med. 309:518, 1983.
11. Okada, R.D., Pohost, G.M. and Kirschenbaum, H.D. N. Engl. J. Med. 301:569, 1979.
12. Wieshammer, S., Delagardella, C., Sigel, H.A., et al. Br. Heart J. 53:603, 1985.
13. Opherk, D., Zebe, H., Werhe, E., et al. Circulation 63:817, 1981.
14. Cannon, R.O., Bonow, R.O., Bacharach, S.L., et al. Circulation 68(Supp III):164, 1983.
15. Legrand, V., Hodgson, J.McB., Bates, E.R., et al. J. Am. Coll. Cardiol. 6:1245, 1985.
16. Vogel, R., LeFree, M., Bates, E., O'Neill, W., Foster, R., Kirlin, P., Smith, D. and Pitt, B. Am. Heart J. 107:153-164, 1984.
17. Bateman, T., Gray, R., Rozanski, A., et al. J. Am. Coll. Cardiol. 1:654, 1983.
18. Bateman, T., Gray, R., Rozanski, A., et al. Circulation 68(Supp III):138, 1983.
19. Ganz, P., Gazpar, J., Barry, W.H., et al. Circulation 68(Supp III):164, 1983.
20. Detre, K.M., Wright, E., Murphy, M.L. and Takaro, T. Circulation 53:627-632, 1976.
21. Fisher, L.K., Judkins, M.P., Lesperance, J., et al. Cath. Cardiovasc. Diagn. 8:565, 1982.
22. Jones, R.H., Floyd, R.D., Austin, E.H., et al. Ann. Surg. 197:743, 1983.

23. Pamelia, F.X., Gibson, R.S., Watson, D.D., et al. Am. J. Cardiol. 55:920, 1985.
24. Habibi, H., Ruddy, P.C., Spencer, R.A., et al. J. Nucl. Med. 28 Supplement A:643, 1987.
25. Johnson, S.H., Bigelow, C. and Lee, K.L. Circulation 74(Supp II):512, 1986.
26. Kotler, T.S., Maddahi, J., Berman, D.S., et al. Circulation 74(Supp II):512, 1986.
27. Bonow. R.O., Kent, K.M., Rosing, D.R., et al. N. Engl. J. Med. 311:1339, 1984.
28. Caralis, D.G., Bailey, I., Kennedy, H.L. and Pitt, B. Br. Heart J. 42:562-567, 1979.
29. Uhl, G.S., Kay, T.N. and Hickman, J.R., Jr. Am. J. Cardiol. 48:1037-43, 1981.
30. Kiat, H., Maddahi, J., Daley, N., Ostrzega, E. and Van Train, K. Circulation 76(Supp IV):1929, 1987.
31. Deanfield, J.E., Shea, M., Kensett, M., Horlock, P., Wilson, R.A., de Landsheere, C.M. and Selwyn, A.P. Lancet 2(8410):1001-5, 1984.
32. Hecht, H.S., Andreae, G. and Chin, H. Circulation 76(Supp IV):1930, 1987.
33. Hakki, A.H., Heo, J. and Iskandrian, A.S. Circuation 76(Supp IV):1943, 1987.
34. Deanfield, J.E., Shea, M.J., Wilson, R.A., Horlock, P., de Landsheere, C.M. and Selwyn, A.P. Am. J. Cardiol. 57:1005-1009, 1986.
35. Assey, M.E., Walters, G.L., Hendrix, G.H., Carabello, B.A., Usher, B.W. and Spann, J.F., Jr. Am. J. Cardiol. 59:497-500, 1987.
36. Cohn, P.F., Brown, E.J., Jr., Swinford, R. and Atkins, H.L. Am. J. Cardiol. 57:521-526, 1986.

DISCUSSION - 2

Dr. Moore: Why do you think we have ST depressions without any coronary artery disease? Do you think that these are some patients that actually have ischemia where you cannot easily detect it with radionucleotide studies? Why do we have false negative and positive ST depressions?

Dr. Kennedy: Dr. Pitt was defining the syndrome X and I keep saying how can I see 5000 coronary artery disease patients coming through our cath lab and no diagnosis of syndrome X in my cath lab. That is because my patients come in, they have chest pain, or they may have a positive ST segment change on their exercise test or on their Holter or any ECG parameter, but their coronary anatomy is normal. We physicians aren't too sensitized to that. Now what percent of the population that is I expect to be small. It is in abnormality of the capillary bed or of the subendocardial layer and I actually think that also occurs somewhat in hypertrophy, but to my knowledge this has not been studied extensively in LVH. Now that accounts for some of the ST false positives. I also know that autonomic changes may affect flow. That interaction of autonomic change and flow reserve has to be looked at. In addition, having an interest in arrhythmia we are all aware that electrolytes change repolarization and so electrolyte imbalance can also alter that. Those are the things we know about. There are probably a lot of things we don't know as well.

Dr. Pitt: On the patient you propose who had a negative radionucleotide test and a positive ECG, I think to my knowledge that is a false positive and probably is due to some repolarization electrolyte changes and I think there is lots of evidence for that. I think a positive exercise ECG and normal anatomy, for the most part do very well and I think that if there isn't some other evidence of ischemia, I really don't think that one can call these people ischemic even though they had ischemic ECG changes and I think they are true false positives.

Dr. Moore: Do you think it would be useful in these patients who have ST segment changes with no angina to do signal averaging? This is a technique that has received a lot of recognition recently where you can do signal averaging and look at the presence of low level late potentials. This is a non-invasive, very cheap procedure to do. It does predict patients who are going to have VT. It does a pretty good job of predicting those. How useful do you really think signal averaging and identifying late potentials are?

Dr. Kennedy: I have been trying to do that for 6 months. Have you tried to do that in a cath lab. Everything has to be grounded, you have to get the balloons in the right place. This is awkward technically right now and now that we have our signal averaging machines that are isolated form electrical sources, they are more portable. We have been working with 12 lead ECG signal averaging and so from that point of view, I think it may offer promise, but we are in an early stage of that. I am looking at that.

Dr. Morganroth: Let's say that I was going to want to study drug X in silent ischemia and I wanted to see if in a placebo controlled trial, drug X suppressed more silent ischemic episodes than placebo, what is the minimum duration of silent ischemia on Holter monitoring necessary to enter such a patient into that trial remembering the variability issue? Should that trial use exercise testing in addition to Holter monitoring or is just Holter monitoring alone sufficient? Should one have a radionuclide test to back up what that ST segment depression might mean on Holter monitoring on exercise testing. Let's assume the study population is the asymptomatic post-infarction patient. I know that there is no data to be certain of each of those.

Dr. Kennedy: Let's go to the last question first. Let's decide if we are going to accept the fact that in a post-MI patient on Holter, that the ST segment change we see is most likely representative of ischemia. As a matter of fact, on our Holter request form that we now employ, when one does a Holter, they have to establish if there is documented evidence of a myocardial infarction on every Holter request we actually have a copy of the 12 lead ECG now to help us in that diagnosis. Number one, I don't feel in that pre-test likelihood I need a second sequential test. If it was an asymptomatic person I would, but this is a person who you know.

Dr. Morganroth: So no radionuclide first?

Dr. Kennedy: No. My post-test likelihood that that represents ischemia from the data of my colleagues gives me assurance that most likely it does. Second question, what is the minimal amount of episodes that one needs to require to establish measures of variability? I know Andrew Selwyn presently is investigating that issue. Shlomo Stern submitted a manuscript on variability and these issues are just now being addressed. The early studies that were done by Drs. Selwyn, Deanfield and Stern have looked at when they take a population, examine the electrocardiographic abnormality, they have required a minimal of so many episodes per week. Most of the studies have been a minimal of 5 episodes per week. That does not answer your question. It has not been definitively answered.

Dr. Morganroth: I was convinced that the variability data shown for select ischemia was identical to arrhythmias. An 80% or greater suppression in the silent ischemic episodes suggests a therapeutic effect rather than spontaneous variability.

Dr. Kennedy: I am a little concerned about that because if they did that study exactly like taking the patients off all their drugs, putting the electrodes in exactly the right place, I am wondering about the selection biases. You have to realize that we have to define that in the variability. Given that, and you and I see all the difficulties there, we are going to do that work and it is going to be defined.

If patients do not have exercised induced situations, why put on a Holter? In other words the implication is that potentially inducible ischemia must be there before one sees spontaneous. The implication is that doing an exercise test if it was negative, you would not see spontaneous episodes. I don't know how true that is over all populations. I think that is another question that has to be defined.

Dr. Morganroth: Don, would you do the exercise test as well as a Holter monitor?

Dr. Weiner: My bias is if you do propose a new drug trial, I think the exercise test is a standard method of assessing new drugs, and there may be different mechanisms involved in ST depression during exercise than during ambulatory monitoring. I think that both procedures are important and I think that both may tell us different things. I think that new drugs should be evaluated to determine whether they lessen both ischemia during exercise testing and during ambulatory monitoring. They may or may not do both and that would be my approach to do both tests.

Dr. Moore: So what you are basically saying is that it is not basically worthwhile. A patient that is going in for his annual physical after 50 years old, they want to do an exercise stress test on you, but if a 12 lead ECG has no indication that you need it, then perhaps you are just wasting that patient's money.

Dr. Kennedy: I don't think ambulatory ECG's should be employed as the primary ECG test for silent ischemia at this point. I feel that it should be an exercise test. I have concerns that the exercise test is showing me potentially inducible ischemia, but I am going on some data and it needs to be studied some more, that most commonly, spontaneous occurring events will not occur in the absence of the potentially inducible. I feel that we investigators have to assure and verify this in larger and broader population groups, but I feel that the exercise test should be the primary ECG mode of looking for ischemia.

Dr. Cohn: I would like to make a comment that in terms of syndrome X while it is of interest academically, I think we should be aware of the fact that the survival within syndrome X is almost the same as in normal individuals. I don't think it is a topic aside from our academic interest that should concern us too much in this kind of setting. Whatever is wrong with these particular individuals and why they have these electrocardiographic changes, it doesn't seem to affect their life span without obstructive disease to the large coronaries.

Dr. Pitt: I think that is certainly true. They have an excellent life span. The only reason for bringing it up is that the true sensitivity of thallium is probably much greater than we think because some of those so-called false positive really have ischemia and the prognosis in the patient who has ischemia and normal coronary arteries is very different than the prognosis in the patient who has ischemia and a significant coronary artery lesion. That doesn't mean that the patient with normal coronary arteries doesn't have ischemia and it doesn't mean that it is not important to know because therapeutically. I think it would still have some meaning that that patient probably should be treated to relieve his symptoms and there is specific treatment to do that rather than someone with just atypical chest pain who doesn't have ischemia.

Dr. Cohn: If we are talking about silent syndrome X then the question comes up should you be treating someone who doesn't have symptoms for disease, it doesn't affect them. I think it is sort of a red herring, though I think it is obviously an important issue from a physiologic point of view. The question I had for Don Weiner was that with the new data he present to Don is actually very similar to the data that has been presented before showing a similar life expectancy and the people without ischemia and with ischemia, except you subdivide and are now looking at MI's and sudden death. The big difference is that in your three vessel disease group, you show data that suggests for the first time as far as I know that the people who have three vessel disease and silent ischemia significantly do worse than those with three vessel disease and angina, which is a very important finding and your numbers I think are adequate enough to make that in the CASS registry, how do you explain this?

Dr. Weiner: I don't know. There was a slight difference but surely not approaching statistical significance of event free rate in patients with silent ischemia versus those with angina and symptomatic ischemia but it appears among patients with three vessel disease that there does seem to be a significant difference, very statistically significant and I really can't explain why, because they are matched for the amount of coronary artery disease. I will have to look to see whether the LV function is equal but I suspect it probably will be between the two groups.

Dr. Cohn: This is one of the uses that you could see where the Holter might be useful because it is possible that within this group even though the two groups have three vessel disease and positive exercise tests, it is possible that one group actually has more out of hospital ischemia than the other and this is one of the reasons that the Holter can be used for risk stratification and hopefully will be in the future.

Dr. Kennedy: I would make a comment about the technology and what is happening here at the end of 1987. I just say to many of the practical people treating patients as well as to pharmaceutical companies assessing things that this silent ischemia, we're like we were when we started with arrhythmia, when all the arrhythmias were all mixed together. We got total ischemia mixed together here and we had to sort out non-sustained V-tach and sustained V-tach, we are having the same situation here. We are sorting out potentially inducible ischemia. We are sorting out spontaneously occurring ischemia and then we are going to arrive upon methods that quantitate it hourly and that is the brink of the threshold we are at right now, this past 3 month period. Major technological advances have come where we are going to be able to quantitate reliably episodes of onset, time frames, minutes of duration, and how that quantity occurs in an hour. Once we get this quantitation with a more precise handle on reliability, then we are going to be able to see which of these parameters of ischemia over a 24 hour day are the most predictive. Physicians make observations. After they make observations on an anecdotal or small basis, then they do limited clinical studies and then we get a data pool and then we develop methods to reliably quantitate it and then we learn to apply the methods correctly in a standardized method and then we do clinical trials. I am very happy about the arrhythmia story because I think it is my guideline to what to do about ischemia here. I feel that we are in a stage right now, particularly in the methodology and the understanding and sorting out these forms of ischemia that we are at the right place. We don't want to run too quickly. We have to do this middle part of defining technology and studies and concepts.

Dr. Weiner: I would like to make also one comment in the next session there is going to be a discussion about drug trials that I would actually like to know from people involved with the FDA would they start to accept end points of ischemic ST depression without angina as an eligibility criteria for admission into a drug trial.

Dr. Lipicky: We do now.

Dr. Weiner: In all trials?

Dr. Lipicky: Certainly, but why do you think we don't yet.

Dr. Weiner: It is my impression having done a lot of drug trials in the past few years that the criteria that we have had to accept were patients who had both angina and ST depression during exercise testing is 5 episodes.

Dr. Lipicky: Certainly not from our lips.

Dr. Weiner: It is good to know that.

Dr. Temple: It must depend upon what you are trying to do with it. For the demonstration that the agent has an anti-ischemic effect, then you probably wouldn't, but if you never showed that angina was improved, you wouldn't have a claim for angina. I mean sooner or later, you have to treat angina, according to our guidelines. Isn't that the way it reads?

Dr. Wiener: Are there any drugs that are approved for ischemia but not angina?

Dr. Lipicky: No, but that certainly is true that if one wants to make a claim for relief of pain, people have to have angina, and if they want to at the same time demonstrate that there is an anti-ischemic effect in the same test, it would be nice to enroll people who have ST segment depression. I understand. If one wants to document an anti-ischemic effect for documentation of the anti-ischemic effect, there is no necessity to have angina as part of the thing that is being measured, never has.

Dr. Temple: That is not what they really want to know. They want to know can you get a pure ischemia claim and the answer is that no one has ever asked us for one for starters and it seems to me that we need to discuss whether that is a meaningful claim.

Dr. Lipicky: Let's talk about that if that is the question. The question is can people get into a trial who have only ST segment changes the answer is yes.

Dr. Temple: They can get into a trial but what will you get out of the trial. What will you have won if you win?

Dr. Lipicky: That wasn't the question asked.

Dr. Temple: This is going to come up a fair amount tomorrow, but the current guideline is for angina, so that the people who enter into the major effectiveness trials are people with angina. Up until now at least, perhaps that will change, no one has come forward with a claim, we relieve ischemia only, and I'm not going to tell you what we do about chest pain because chest pain doesn't matter, the only important thing is relieving ischemia. That up until now has not been a claim. There was some discussion this morning whether that should be a claim and that is a fair question, but really that hasn't been addressed. The guideline also says that to be an anti-anginal agent, you can't just be an analgesic. You have to treat the angina by relieving its cause which is ischemia so you have to show both and there is no particular reason why you couldn't show one in one study and one in the other, so that is what Ray's answer is , I think about the first part.

Dr. Lipicky: But really I guess there is more to it than that. If one is looking at the current attitudinal set that goes into the considerations with respect to an anti-anginal agent the set is that it is for symptomatic care and that therefore there needs to be a symptom that would lead to the claim because it is for the symptomatic care. The attitudinal set is such because it isn't clear that there is a benefit or there is no clear demonstration of benefit from anything other than having the symptom treated.

Dr. Moore: Ray, if it improves quality of life, is that enough?

Dr. Lipicky: Sure. But now, what it also says is that there has to be an anti-ischemic effect and if one is attempting to demonstrate and anti-ischemic effect, to support the claim of having symptomatic benefits in patients with coronary artery disease, than indeed one can enroll patients with ST segment depression only and the measurement of pain becomes a non-significant end point.

Dr. Pepine: I would like to carry on where we left off. The guidelines, at least the guidelines I have been presented, have pain right on top, pain and nitroglycerine pill counts. Now the problem that I see in this whole thing is that industry or the scientific community develops these compounds or devices in animals. Animals don't have pain. They all have anti-ischemic properties and we get a wealth of data and we show that these drugs or devices are tremendous anti-ischemic drugs and then we forget and go to the clinic because we are stuck with anti-anginal issues, and then in the clinic in order to comply with variability issues, in the trade we call it FDA angina. We go and screen 100's of patients to get 10 that comply with your requirements, to have enough, less variability, etc. and then we force those poor patients into walking on a treadmill so that their effort tolerance is improved by your primary measurement as timed onset of angina. Then we take all of that and if it applies in a couple of trials, we have our two positive trials and we say, good, anti-anginal issue, but what do we really do. I mean we relieve pain in a small number of people, we really don't know anything about ischemia because we forgot all that information that was dropped along the way because we didn't have a prime area ischemic indication. So that is where we have to change the thinking. I am not blaming you for it, I am not saying you are responsible for perpetuating it. I am saying, let's look at it from a different point of view, from the ischemic point of view. If you look at it from that point of view, pain will fall by the wayside, pain that is related to ischemia will go away. It will disappear. I think that that is where the focus has to be, on the front end of ischemia, not on the pain.

Dr. Temple: The trouble is, it seems to me, how would you define the amount of relief in ischemia for example in a trial for example in which there was no pain end point, that represented a meaningful improvement for the patient's anginal syndrome. How would you link those two if you didn't study pain?

Dr. Pepine: I could use the definition you use for angina, 50% reduction if I wanted to pull one out of the sky, I could use the definition of eliminating all ischemia. I could say we could only eliminate high risk ischemia. Don Weiner gave you a beautiful list of markers of high risk ischemia and other people have done the same thing. We have a lot of fairly objective end points that are much better than a 50% reduction in angina.

Dr. Temple: Are you arguing that these would be perfectly suitable ways of knowing that the drug is anti-anginal or are you saying that we now know that we will improve the survival of these people.

Dr. Pepine: I didn't say either one of those two.

Dr. Temple: Then why are we doing this?

Dr. Pepine: We would know that the drug was anti-ischemia. I say that before you get to first base in ischemic heart disease, you have to have an anti-ischemic agent, like you have to have an anti-hypertensive agent or an antiarrhythmic agent, or you can't go anywhere. We wouldn't have gone anywhere if we had had an anti-headache agent to treat blood pressure and that is what we are doing. We have anti-chest pain agents and in most of those patients we don't know whether or not they have ischemic heart disease.

Dr. Temple: The current standards anyway, and this has been emphasized by the re-write of them, is that the treatment of angina is supposed to be with agents that relieve ischemia. So you measure the effect on the anginal syndrome, principally by exercise testing, I should say, not by anginal counts anymore, and simultaneously show that you have improved ischemia. So it is not that the second of those end points is being missed. What is true is at the moment at least, we have not accepted, and have not been asked to accept the claim that didn't come with some evidence that the anginal syndrome, the pain itself was not relieved and we got a very strong message from the advisory committee that for an anginal drug, you need to improve pain. They thought it was an entirely separate question as to whether one might have a drug which was intended to treat ischemia independent whether it had any relationship to angina and the discussion this morning focused to some extent on why you would want to do that exactly. What were you think you were doing when you did that? Would you be improving survival? Would you be relieving the transient periods of abnormal ventricular function that may have some impact or what would you be doing when you did that and how would you lay those effects which you have never measured or known off against the side effects of these drugs which they all have. For what it is worth, it seems to me that when you don't know what your ultimate effect is, when you are not relieving something that is bothering the patient or altering his survival, you don't really know how to deal with questions of small changes in lipids and all those kinds of things. To me the treatment of hypertension indicates some degree of caution. We don't know why most hypertension studies have not shown improvement in the coronary artery disease end points, but it seems like one possibility at least is that the effect is rather small and is overcome by some of the abnormal effects on lipids or potassium or who knows what, that some of the anti-hypertensive drugs give you. If you are looking here at changes that you can't measure, haven't really measured yet, it seems to me you are in a very difficult position as to whether you are having a favorable impact on such things as survival which must be the main reason for treating silent and non-symptomatic ischemia.

III. TRIAL DESIGNS

9

LONGITUDINAL (NATURAL HISTORY) STUDIES OF SILENT MYOCARDIAL ISCHEMIA

J. THOMAS BIGGER JR., M.D., and THE MSSMI INVESTIGATORS

Department of Medicine, Columbia University, New York, New York
and the Arrhythmia Control Unit, Columbia-Presbyterian Medical Center
630 West 168th Street, New York, New York 10032

ASYMPTOMATIC ST DEPRESSION DURING HOLTER RECORDINGS

It is known that about 25% of myocardial infarctions occur without associated pain (1). Recent reports of unsuspected, frequent and prolonged episodes of asymptomatic ST depression (ASTD) during Holter recordings made in patients with clinical angina pectoris and positive exercise tests have raised important issues for the evaluation and treatment of coronary disease. The traditional role of angina as the best indicator of myocardial ischemia may have to be reevaluated, since several studies have shown that ASTD occurs more frequently than symptomatic ischemia in many patients with coronary disease (2-11). Atrial pacing in patients with angina pectoris shows that angina is a relatively late event during myocardial ischemia (12). If ASTD reflects clinically meaningful ischemia, then overt angina represents only 25% of the total ischemic burden. Moreover, incomplete data suggest than an increased and clinically unsuspected risk may be conferred on patients who have frequent episodes of ASTD (13,14).

While episodes of ASTD are of great interest in the understanding of coronary disease, documenting them is of little value unless they indicate increased risk. Several studies have considered prognosis in patients with ASTD; but these studies are almost entirely of small numbers, not designed for follow-up, with inadequate design and insufficient end-points (2-11,13,14). Other investigations employed treadmill tests, and they offer little evidence that ambulatory monitoring of ASTD is useful for evaluating prognosis. Thus, drug studies for eliminating ASTD are premature until the risk of ASTD is defined.

A number of important investigations indicate that properly recorded ST depressions on the Holter do represent episodes of myocardial ischemia (9,15). These recordings have shown that myocardial ischemia is common during daily activity, even in the absence of angina or other symptoms, suggesting that ischemia may be caused by spasm or by transient platelet aggregations or thrombi. Whether we should ignore these episodes of ASTD or actively intervene with treatment cannot be answered at this time. To address the significance of ASTD, we have planned the Multicenter Study of Silent Myocardial Ischemia (MSSMI), a prospective study to determine if ASTD can predict clinically significant adverse cardiac events in patients with coronary occlusive disease.

EXPERIMENTAL DESIGN AND METHODS

General Objective

The major goal of MSSMI is to determine if ST depression detected by Holter recordings (so-called silent ischemia) in patients recently hospitalized for an acute coronary ischemic event identifies a subgroup at increased risk of subsequent cardiac mortality and morbidity events.

TIMETABLE FOR
MULTICENTER STUDY OF SILENT MYOCARDIAL ISCHEMIA

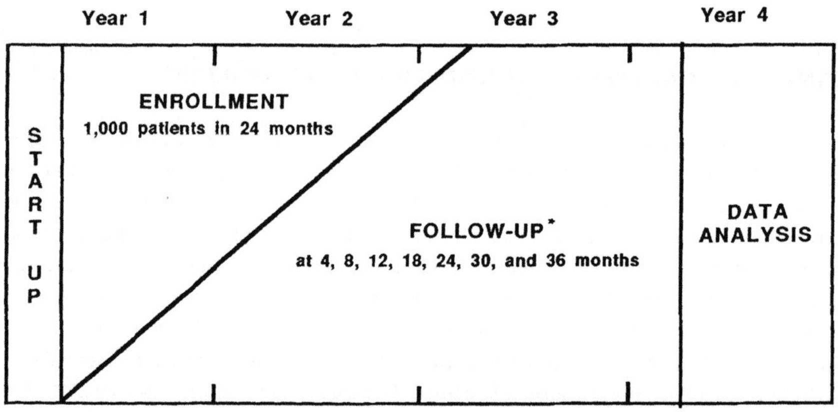

*Patients will be followed 12 to 36 months (24 months average)

Chronologic Phases

MSSMI has three phases: (1) planning and start-up, (2) enrollment and follow-up, and (3) data analysis (see Figure 1). The start-up phase will last 3 months. During this period, personnel will be trained in recruitment and data acquisition. About 1,000 patients will be enrolled during a 24-month period. These patients will be followed for a minimum of one year to a maximum of three years with follow-up contact every 4 to 6 months. The vital status (alive or dead) of non-participants will be determined one year after such patients decline participation. For the 1,000 enrolled patients, prospectively defined fatal and non-fatal cardiac end points will be characterized and recorded during 12-36 months of follow-up. Prior hospital data and baseline clinical information will be recorded on the patients at the time of enrollment

(2-6 months after the index coronary event). Special studies, including a 24-hour Holter recording, a Bruce protocol exercise test, and a thallium perfusion scan, will be obtained on all enrolled patients during a one-week period. The analysis phase will last 9 months. Data analysis will be carried out to evaluate prospectively specified primary, secondary, and tertiary hypotheses. The significance of the results will be evaluated, external criticism and review will be solicited, and manuscripts will be prepared.

Sample Size Calculation

Computation of the sample size required for this study was based on: (1) the primary objective of the study; (2) estimated proportion of patients with asymptomatic ST depression (ASTD); (3) estimated combined mortality and morbidity event rates; (4) the selection of a relative risk that is clinically worth detecting for those with ASTD compared to those without ASTD; and (5) a one-tailed test of significance.

Our primary objective is to determine if asymptomatic ST depression (ASTD) is associated with a significantly increased cardiac event rate during 2-year follow-up when compared to that of patients without ASTD. Based upon our own pilot studies and a variety of reports in the literature (1-14), we estimated that: (1) the proportion of patients with ASTD will be between 0.20 and 0.30; (2) the overall population event rate will be between 10% and 20% in two years; and (3) we believe it would be important to detect a relative risk of 1.5 or greater in those with ASTD. We reasoned that it is appropriate to utilize a one-tailed test of significance in our sample size calculation because we are testing a one-sided hypothesis that ASTD confers risk. We are not testing the alternate hypothesis, i.e., that ASTD confers benefit and is associated with a reduced event rate with a relative risk less than 1.0.

With these estimates and assumptions, we can construct the following table:

	Estimated Proportion of Enrolled	Estimated 2-year Cardiac Event Rate
ASTD Present	0.20 - 0.30	19 - 22%
ASTD Absent	0.70 - 0.80	12 - 14%
Total	1.0	13 -16%

Assuming an ASTD proportion of 0.25 and a population event rate of 15% (alpha = 0.05, one-tailed), approximately 1,000 patients would provide enough power (>80%) to detect a relative risk of 1.5 (e.g., 20% vs. 13%) in the 2-year event rates for those with and without ASTD.

Enrollment and Follow-up

During the enrollment period, each participating hospital will maintain an accurate log of patients admitted to its coronary care and stepdown/telemetry units to indicate whether or not each patient is eligible. All eligible patients will be contacted prior to hospital discharge regarding possible enrollment in MSSMI beginning 2-6 months after their CCU or stepdown/telemetry unit admission for their index event.

Patient eligibility. Patients who satisfy *all* of the following criteria will be eligible for enrollment: (1) admission to a coronary care or stepdown/telemetry unit of a hospital affiliated with the 12 enrolling centers, (2) male or female less than 76 years of age on the day of hospital admission, (3) an acute coronary ischemic event prompting hospitalization, (4) residency within a 30 mile radius of the enrolling center, and (5) survival for 2 to 6 months after index hospitalization. The ischemic event must be: (a) definite acute myocardial infarction - meet strict MSSMI enzyme definition together with symptoms and/or ECG changes consistent with an acute coronary event; (b) unstable non-infarction angina - requires an increase in the frequency and/or duration of typical anginal symptoms or the new development of angina at rest with transient ischemic ECG changes (ST-segment elevation or depression of 1 mm or more, or T-wave inversion or pseudonormalization) without enzyme elevation indicative of infarction, and (c) myocardial ischemic-related left ventricular dysfunction and/or increased ventricular irritability (by strict definitions in the MSSMI operations manual).

Exclusion criteria. The following conditions will exclude otherwise eligible patients: (1) coronary artery bypass graft surgery between the index hospital admission and the enrollment window 2 to 6 months later; (2) coronary angioplasty performed less than 2 months before the 2 to 6 month window of enrollment; (3) significant co-morbidity such as malignancy or severe hepatic, renal, or cerebral disease; (4) musculo-skeletal disorders which would prevent the patient from taking the exercise thallium study; (5) failure of the patient to agree to take both special studies (24-hour Holter recording and the exercise thallium study); (6) receiving treatment with a cardiac glycoside; (7) left or right bundle branch block pattern or atrial fibrillation on the ECG at enrollment; (8) implanted pacemaker; (9) participation in another investigational study; and (10) pregnant women.

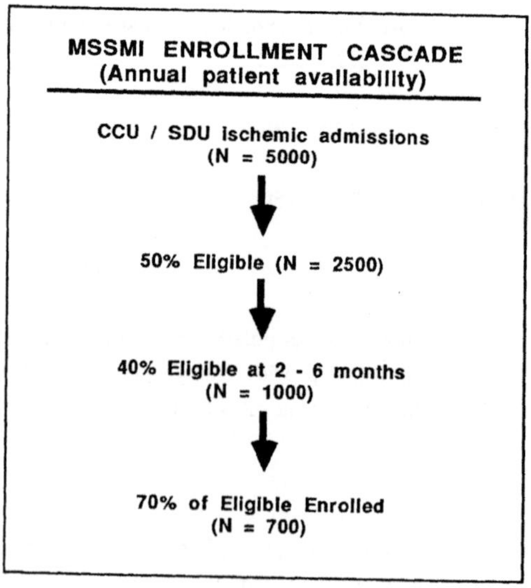

Enrollment cascade: Patients will be enrolled from 15 or 16 participating hospitals. The CCU and stepdown/telemetry unit registries of each of the participating hospitals during the first 6 months of 1986 were reviewed and indicated that about 5000 patients per year will meet our criteria for acute coronary ischemic events. We estimate that about 50% of these patients will meet our eligibility criteria, i.e., about 2,500 patients per year. We expect about 40% will still be eligible 2 to 6 months later, about 1,000, and that about 70% or 700 patients will enroll in the MSSMI (Figure 2).

Patient Recruitment. We will request permission of a personal physician to approach his/her patient for enrollment as soon as it is clear that the patient is likely to meet the eligibility criteria. If the primary physician agrees, the patient will be contacted prior to hospital discharge and informed of the study. If the patient is favorably inclined, the patient's name, address, and phone number will be recorded so that he/she can be contacted again 2 to 6 months later for formal enrollment. At that time, the study will again be explained to the patient and the special study tests (24-hour Holter and the exercise thallium study) described. The patient will be enrolled in the study when he or she signs the consent for participation. Patients who refuse to participate (non-enrollment) will be identified and a record kept so that their ultimate survival status can be ascertained one year later.

Baseline data collection. Patients will be enrolled 2-6 months after index cardiac event. Formal enrollment initiates the collection of data - retrospective information from the index hospitalization and baseline clinical information on the day of enrollment (16). The study coordinator will interview and examine the patient and record the information on data forms. A baseline 12-lead ECG will be recorded at this time and forwarded to the ECG Core Laboratory for interpretation (17). Two non-invasive special studies will be obtained within one week of enrollment that should provide relevant information about overt and silent myocardial ischemia: (1) a 24-hour continuous ECG recording, and (2) an exercise thallium study. The information from these special tests will be analyzed in core laboratories and used as predictor variables to determine whether silent myocardial ischemia is associated with an increased incidence of cardiac ischemic events.

24-hour Holter tape recorders. Marquette model 8500 cassette tape recorders will be used at all centers participating in the study. The frequency characteristics of the recorders will be tested and validated at Marquette Medical Electronics, Inc. before distribution to the Holter Core Laboratory. The Marquette recorders will be tested for overshoot, droop, and phase distortion in the Holter Core Laboratory at Columbia University. Also, the recorders will be checked to ensure a gain of 1,000X.

Diary and activity. Holter ECG recordings will always begin on a weekday morning. A recorder will be placed on the patient and he/she will be asked to perform all of his/her regular activities and to describe them in a diary. The instructions for use of the diary are part of the operations manual for the study, and each technician or study coordinator that applies Holter recorders will be trained to instruct patients to record the activity level and the character and intensity of angina pectoris or possible anginal equivalents in the diary (16), for a future analysis of the correlation between symptoms or physical activity and the ECG findings. Postural and respiratory maneuvers will be a routine part of the hook-up procedure. The patient will lie down for one minute, sit down for one minute and then stand for one minute. Each patient will be asked to hyperventilate for a period of 30 seconds. These postural and respiratory maneuvers will be bracketed on the tape by 1 mV calibration pulses so that the Holter Core Laboratory can identify them. A strip of each ECG lead and the 1 mV calibration pulses will be made using an ECG machine. These strips will be sent to the Holter Core Laboratory along with the Holter cassette and diary.

Medications. On the day of recording, the patients will take their prescribed medications, including beta blockers, calcium channel blockers, or nitrates. If chest pain occurs during the recording, patients will be allowed to use anti-ischemic medications as prescribed by their primary physicians, e.g., sublingual nitroglycerin. The time of medication use, especially sublingual nitroglycerin or isosorbide dinitrate, will be recorded in the diary.

Analysis of 24-hour ECG recordings. All tapes will be analyzed at the Holter Core Laboratory at Columbia University using the Marquette 8100 Holter analysis system running version 5.x software with some special enhancements for ST segment analysis. The following information will be recorded on each episode of ST depression.

1. Start time (the time when ST segment first shows >1 mm [0.1 mV] depression referenced to the resting ST baseline).

2. Stop time (the time when the ST segment returns to within 1 mm of baseline).

3. The maximum ST depression during the episode, measured in mm.

4. The integral of ST depression, i.e., the sum of the instantaneous ST levels during the ischemic episode, referenced to the baseline.

5. Heart rate at the following times: 1 minute before, at the onset of the episode of ST depression, at the time of maximum heart rate during the ischemic episode, at the time of maximum ST depression, and 1 minute after the end of the ischemic episode.

6. The number of ventricular premature depolarizations (VPD) occurring during the episode.

A 6 sec strip of ECG will be taken at the time of maximum ST depression for each ischemic episode. Also, a 6 sec ECG strip will be taken 1 min before and 1 min after each ischemic episode. The Marquette 8100 system will be programmed to write a 10 sec ECG strip every hour during the 24-hour recording as a check on undetected ischemic episodes in the recording. In addition to the ECG strips, the following trend plots and tables will be made available for review by the cardiologist.

1. A high resolution ST table that gives the median ST depression or elevation in tenths of a mm every 15 sec throughout the 24-hour recording.

2. A high resolution ST elevation/depression graphic trend plot.

3. A heart rate trend plot on the same time scale as the ST trend so that ST elevation or depression and the corresponding heart rate can be visually correlated.

4. A plot of VPD frequency as a function of time on the same scale as the ST changes and heart rate to evaluate whether ventricular arrhythmias are more common during periods of ischemia compared to other times during the recording.

The measurements made above will permit us to ascertain whether or not ST segment depression occurred in a recording. The minimum criteria for an ischemic episode will be *1 mm of ST depression that persists for at least one minute,* a commonly used definition. If less than one minute separates two periods of significant ischemia as determined by the definition given above, then the two episodes will be combined. Also, we will count the number of ischemic episodes in positive tapes and determine the duration of each ischemic episode. The maximum ST depression, the magnitude of ST depression as a function of time, the total ischemic time, and the ST depression-time integral will be measured and coded in the database. Also, the relationship of the ischemic episodes to heart rate changes and ventricular arrhythmias will be coded along with the number of VPD during a control period with identical heart rate. The matched pairs of counts (ischemia versus control) of total VPD, paired VPD, and episodes of ventricular tachycardia will be accumulated in the database at the Coordination and Data Center. These data will permit a definite answer to questions about the relationships between the presence, duration or severity of spontaneous ASTD and the presence, frequency and repetitiveness of ventricular arrhythmias adjusting for time of day and heart rate. Similar methodology will permit automated data collection on the time course of heart rate during ischemic episodes and on the relationship between magnitude of heart rate change and magnitude of ST depression.

Exercise thallium study. The exercise thallium study consists of a Bruce-protocol exercise test and a thallium perfusion scan (18-22). Three exercise leads, aVf, V3, and V5, will be obtained pre-exercise (supine, sitting, standing, and with hyperventilation), every minute during exercise, at peak exercise, and 1 minute after exercise. Supine 12-lead recordings will be taken at 3 and 6 minutes following exercise. The exercise test will be evaluated in terms of duration, symptoms, hemodynamics, arrhythmia, and ischemia (ST-T change). The pertinent ECG recordings together with heart rate, blood pressure, and symptom occurrence information will be forward to the Exercise Core Laboratory at Highland Hospital, Rochester, New York. At the peak of exercise, 2.0 mCi of 201-Tl will be administered intravenously and the patient will continue to exercise for an additional 30-60 sec. With the patient in the supine position, imaging will begin at 5 minutes after injection in the 40° left anterior oblique, followed by the left lateral and anterior projections. All images will be recorded for 10 minutes using a standard gamma camera interfaced to a dedicated computer. The three views will be repeated at 3 to 4 hours after 201-Tl administration. Particular care will be taken to carefully reproduce the initial positioning. Images will be collected in a 64 x 64 matrix. Each individual enrolling center will use a quantitative analysis technique based on similar concepts. The essence is their use of an interpolative background technique (18-22). To enhance uniformity between enrolling centers, quantitation will utilize the circumferential as opposed to the horizontal profile. Using this approach counts are displayed for 60-6° angle segments based on the maximal count per pixel.

The redistribution images will be similarly analyzed. Images will be read in the Thallium Core Laboratory at the Long Island Jewish-Hillside Medical Center and 10% will be reread at Yale University.

Clinic follow-up visits. Patients will be seen by the study coordinator every 4 months during the first year, then every 6 months thereafter. Medical/cardiac information will be obtained with regard to interval history including anginal status, diagnostic and therapeutic interventions (coronary angiography, CABG, PTCA, pacemaker, etc.), and hospitalization for cardiac events. Concurrent medications will be recorded. Weight, blood pressure, and heart rate will be obtained. These visits will maintain periodic contact with the patients and will enhance our ability to identify cardiac end points in close proximity to the event. The findings at each follow-up visit will be recorded in follow-up data forms and transmitted to the Coordinating and Data Center (CDC) at the University of Rochester for entry into the data management file.

24-hour Holter ECG recording at the 4-month visit. The purpose of this recording is to provide information about the stability and variability of Holter ASTD at two points in time (baseline and four months). The ambulatory recording will be analyzed at the Holter Core Laboratory (Columbia University).

12-lead ECG at one year and trial termination. The purpose of these recordings is to obtain information on interim silent infarction as demonstrated by new Q wave development since the prior tracing. The ECG will be coded at the ECG Core Laboratory (Roosevelt Hospital, New York City) using the Manhattan Code which is well suited to identify regional Q wave abnormalities and pattern changes in serial recording (17).

End point event data. The prespecified end points in this study are cardiac mortality and cardiac morbidity with rehospitalization due to either myocardial infarction or unstable angina (crescendo angina or angina decubitus). Although we will identify and record CABG and PTCA procedures, these "events" will not be used as end points in the primary analysis because these events represent physician decision as much as disease state. For the purposes of the primary analysis, only one event, the first one to occur (mortality, rehospitalization with myocardial infarction, or rehospitalization with unstable angina) will be used for each patient. Documentation of the cause of death will be based on information collected from witnesses, relatives, death certificates, autopsy reports, and hospital records. The location of death, the underlying cause of death, the chronology of the terminal event will be recorded, and the suspected mechanism of the terminal event will be categorized using the Hinkle classification scheme (23). Whenever a study coordinator at a participating hospital identifies an enrolled patient as having been hospitalized, the hospital record will be reviewed and a MSSMI Rehospitalization Categorization Form completed. An experienced End Point and Events Subcommittee will review and independently classify all mortality and morbidity end points.

Data Analysis

Primary analysis. The primary analysis consists of two parts and will use the entire enrolled population. The first analysis will evaluate the association between a prespecified Holter ischemia variable, e.g., the presence or absence of ST depression >1 mm (0.1 mV) and end point events (cardiac mortality or hospitalization with non-fatal infarction/unstable angina) during the entire follow-up using the Cox proportional hazard model (24). The only covariates in the first Cox regression analysis will be the enrolling centers. Assuming a meaningful association, this same Holter variable will then be studied together with prespecified exercise and thallium perfusion variables as well as a limited number of clinical variables to determine if Holter ASTD makes an independent contribution to the prediction of end point events. The Cox proportional hazards model adjusted for center and other covariates will be utilized with and without adjustment for treatment at the time of baseline testing.

Secondary analyses. Several secondary analyses are planned to further explore: (1) the relationships among Holter ischemia variables (ST depression frequency, magnitude, and duration) and outcome; (2) the interrelationship between several measures of myocardial ischemia; (3) the possible interaction between Holter ASTD and heart rate with respect to outcome; (4) the interrelationships among several Holter recorded variables (ST depression, heart rate, heart rate variability, and ventricular ectopy) and their joint independent contribution to end point events; and (5) the effect of Holter ASTD outcome in various population subgroups such as anterior vs. posterior myocardial infarction, those with and without pre-enrollment coronary angioplasty, and the entry classification groupings (myocardial infarction, unstable angina, ischemic left ventricular dysfunction and/or ischemic arrhythmias).

Tertiary analyses. Lower priority analyses will take place after there has been a considerable exploration of the data base. Some of the planned analyses include: (1) an evaluation of the stability and variability of the Holter-recorded variables (ST depression, heart rate, heart rate variability, and ventricular ectopy frequency) over the 4-month interval between baseline and the first follow-up visit in this relatively stable population; (2) an evaluation of the associations and significance of Holter-recorded ST elevations in this population; (3) the frequency of occurrence of asymptomatic myocardial infarction in this population as determined by the development of new Q waves on ECGs recorded one year after enrollment and at study termination when compared to the baseline tracing; and (4) a detailed descriptive analysis of the changing pattern of therapeutic practices in this well defined population with follow-up every 4 to 6 months over an average of 24 months per patient (25).

Rationale for Specific Decisions

Why the minimum 2-month interval between the index hospitalization and MSSMI enrollment? The main goal of this study is to evaluate the clinical significance of asymptomatic ischemia in a relatively stable population of patients with documented coronary heart disease. Presently, a wide variety of medical and surgical interventions are utilized following hospitalization for an acute cardiac ischemic event. We wanted to study patients whose therapeutic management had been stabilized. Our judgement, experience, and previous research suggest that a plateau of therapeutic and clinical stability is achieved by 2 to 6 months after an index event.

Why have we chosen to exclude patients who have had coronary artery bypass graft surgery (CABG) after their index coronary event? CABG surgery is associated with interruption of some of the neural pathways to and from the heart and with ST and T wave changes secondary to non-ischemic postoperative pericarditis. The inclusion of such patients would potentially confound our study of prevalence and significance of silent myocardial ischemia.

Why have we chosen to include patients who had percutaneous transluminal angioplasty (PTCA) 2 or more months before enrollment? Angioplasty is often used to treat patients who have experienced a significant myocardial ischemic event. The intervention usually is applied to 1 vessel in an attempt to reduce a specific coronary stenosis; the procedure is rarely definitive. Among initially successful cases, recurrent stenosis with requirement for a second procedure is highest during the first few months with relative stabilization thereafter. Unlike the CABG patients, PTCA does not interfere with the appreciation of angina pectoris and does not confound the interpretation of Holter-recorded ST segment changes. By delaying enrollment until two months or more after PTCA, we believe we will be dealing with a relatively stable group of PTCA patients who, for the most part, will still have underlying coronary disease with a potential for silent ischemia and recurrent cardiac events.

Why have we decided to evaluate patients with Holter recordings, exercise tests, and thallium imaging while on their anti-ischemic medications? Patients enrolled in this study are likely to be on varying doses of medications including beta blockers, calcium channel blockers, nitrates and aspirin. Some patients also will be on antiarrhythmic agents, diuretics, vasodilators or other drugs (antihypertensives and hypoglycemic agents) for related conditions. Patients taking digitalis will be excluded from the present study because of the profound effects of cardiac glycosides on ST segment responses. The influence of many of the non-glycoside drugs on Holter-recorded asymptomatic ST depression (ASTD) and other variables is unknown, but these agents are likely to have only modest impact on the interpretation of Holter and exercise ST segment data. Since these agents will tend to suppress both symptoms and ASTD, We considered transient discontinuation of antianginal agents during baseline observations. However, this might cause ischemic problems in some of these outpatients who are recovering from a recent coronary event. In a few individuals, ischemic recurrence could lead to alarming, disabling, costly, and even hazardous consequences. We concluded that temporary discontinuation of antianginal therapy for baseline tests was inappropriate and impractical from a safety standpoint. Furthermore, baseline evaluation of patients off antianginals may have little relevance to outcomes during long-term follow-up with patients on therapy. The policy of evaluation while on antianginal drugs has been adopted by investigators in previous studies without evident impairment of the predictive capacity of exercise thallium tests (26) or Holter ASTD (14).

How will we adjust for the effect of treatment on outcome? Since we will not control for the effects of antianginal drugs in the design, we will make statistical adjustments for them during the analysis. There is no single right way to adjust for the use of medication in a non-randomized study such as this. In the primary analysis of data from non-randomized studies it is important to separate the influence of medical conditions and their associated risk factors from the influence of drugs used to treat these conditions. One approach is to exclude medications from the initial set of risk covariates and examine drug effects on the association between Holter ASTD and cardiac adverse events only after the independent effect of Holter ASTD, adjusted for non-therapeutic risk factors, has been assessed. Thus, the use of various medications such as beta blockers, calcium channel blockers, nitrates, and aspirin, alone and in combination, can be entered into the Cox regression analysis as independent risk factors to evaluate their confounding effect.

Summary

Clinical and laboratory observations reviewed in this conference suggest that asymptomatic ST segment depression on ambulatory Holter ECG recordings may be an important indicator of clinically "silent" myocardial ischemia reflecting advanced and potentially unstable coronary occlusive disease. However, the clinical correlates of ASTD in patients recovered from myocardial infarction or unstable angina are incompletely understood, and the relation of ASTD to long-term prognosis in these patients is unknown. We are undertaking a multicenter study in this patient group utilizing ambulatory 24-hour continuous ECG recordings to determine the frequency, severity, and duration of silent myocardial ischemia occurring during usual daily activities. This information will be analyzed in conjunction with ST segment depression on treadmill exercise, reversible perfusion defects on stress thallium testing, and several prespecified, clinical parameters to evaluate the independent prognostic significance of ASTD.

The *primary objective* of this study is to determine if Holter detected ASTD (silent ischemia) in ambulatory patients with documented coronary heart disease is associated with an increased incidence of overt cardiac events (cardiac death or hospitalization with non-fatal myocardial infarction or unstable angina) during a 1-3 year follow-up period. The primary analysis also will assess whether Holter recorded ASTD adds to prognostic information obtained from routine clinical evaluation and from non-invasive testing that is now in widespread use for evaluation of myocardial ischemia.

Secondary objectives of this study include an evaluation of the interactions and associations between frequency, severity, and duration of Holter ASTD and other ischemic variables derived from exercise electrocardiography and stress thallium imaging. An association of Holter ASTD with exercise-induced ST changes and reversible perfusion defects in thallium uptake on stress testing may identify various ischemic subgroups with different cardiac event rates. Alternatively, our study may disclose overlapping and clinically redundant testing procedures. We plan to evaluate the prognostic risk of Holter ASTD occurring at lower vs. higher heart rates (e.g., cut point 90 beats per min) to obtain insight into suspected vasoactive (supply) and increased myocardial oxygen consumption (demand) mechanisms of silent myocardial ischemia. An additional objective is to determine the interrelationship between ASTD and ventricular arrhythmias on Holter monitoring and to evaluate the association of these combined ischemic and arrhythmic parameters with cardiac mortality and morbidity events.

We hope that the findings of our study will provide insight into the pathophysiologic significance of ASTD and the suitability of this variable as a risk indicator and as a potential target for controlled clinical trials. It is possible that ASTD could serve as a surrogate for ischemic endpoints in clinical trials. Conversely, it may be that ASTD adds nothing to more conventional measures of ischemia, e.g., exercise ST segment depression or temporary perfusion deficit during exercise thallium studies.

MSSMI KEY PERSONNEL

Principal Investigator

Arthur J. Moss, M.D.	University of Rochester	Rochester, NY

MSSMI ENROLLING CENTERS

Co-Principal Investigators	**Hospital**	**City, State**
J. Thomas Bigger, Jr., M.D.	The Presbyterian Hospital	New York, NY
James Coromilas, M.D.		
Robert B. Case, M.D.	St. Luke's Hospital Center	New York, NY
Henry M. Greenberg, M.D.	Roosevelt Hospital Center	New York, NY
Edward M. Dwyer, Jr., M.D.		
Edgar Lichstein, M.D.	Maimonides Medical Center	Brooklyn, NY
John J. Gregory, M.D.	Overlook Hospital	Summit, NJ
John Gillespie, M.D.	Highland Hospital	Rochester, NY
Robert Goldstein, M.D.	Malcolm Grow Air Force Hospital	Bethesda, MD
	Walter Reed Army Hospital	Bethesda, MD
Lucy Van Voorhees, M.D.	Washington Hospital Center	Washington, DC
Frank I. Marcus, M.D.	University Arizona Health Center	Tucson, AZ
	St. Mary's Hospital	Tucson, AZ
John Parker, M.D.	Kingston General Hospital	Kingston, Canada
	Hotel Dieu	Kingston, Canada
Shlomo Stern, M.D.	Bikur Cholim Hospital	Jerusalem, Israel
Dan Tzivoni, M.D.		
Peter J. Schwartz, M.D.	Oespedale Maggiore	Milano, Italia
MSSMI COORDINATION AND DATA CENTER		
Arthur J. Moss, M.D.	University of Rochester	Rochester, NY
MSSMI HOLTER CORE LABORATORY		
J. Thomas Bigger, Jr., M.D.	Columbia University	New York, NY
MSSMI RADIONUCLIDE CORE LABORATORY		
Monty Bodenheimer, M.D.	Long Island Jewish Hillside Medical Center	New Hyde Park, NY
MSSMI ECG READING CENTER		
Henry M. Greenberg, M.D.	Roosevelt Hospital Center	New York, NY
Edward M. Dwyer, Jr., M.D.		
MSSMI EXERCISE TEST CORE LABORATORY		
John Gillespie, M.D.	Highland Hospital	Rochester, NY

REFERENCES

1. Kannel WB, Abbott RD. Incidence and prognosis of unrecognized myocardial infarction. N Engl J Med 1984; 311:1144-1147.

2. Nesto RW, Phillips RT. Asymptomatic myocardial ischemia in diabetic patients. Am J Med 1986; 80(Supp 4C):40-47.

3. Cecchi AC, Dovellini E, Marchi F, Pucci P, Santoro G, Fazzini F. Silent myocardial ischemia during ambulatory electrocardiographic monitoring in patients with effort angina. J AM Coll Cardiol 1983; 1:934-939.

4. Stern S, Tzivoni D. Early detection of silent ischaemic heart disease by 24-hour electrocardiographic monitoring of active subjects. Br Heart J 1974; 36:481-486.

5. Schang SJ, Pepine CJ. Transient asymptomatic S-T segment depression during daily activity. Am J Cardiol 1977; 39:396-402.

6. Cohn PF. Silent myocardial ischemia: to treat or not to treat? Hosp Pract 1983; 125-138.

7. Deanfield JE, Selwyn AP, Chierchia S, Maseri A, Ribiero P, Krikler D. Myocardial ischemia during daily life in patients with stable angina; its relation to heart rate changes. Lancet 1983; 753-758.

8. Chierchia S, Lazzari M, Freedman B, Burnelli C, Maseri A. Impairment of myocardial perfusion and function during painless myocardial ischemia. J Am Coll Cardiol 1983; 1:924-930.

9. Deanfield JE, Shea M, Ribiero P, Landsheere C, Wilson R, Horlock P, Selwyn A. Transient ST-segment depression as a marker of myocardial ischemia during daily life. Am J Cardiol 1984; 54:1195-1200.

10. Biagini A, Mazzei MG, Carpeggiani C, Testa R, Antonelli R, Michelassi C, L'Abbate A, Maseri A. Vasospastic ischemic mechanism of frequent asymptomatic transient ST-T changes during continuous electrocardiographic monitoring in selected unstable patients. Am Heart J 1982; 103:13-20.

11. Deanfield JE, Ribiero P, Oakley K, Krikler D, Selwyn A. Analysis of ST-segment changes in normal subjects: implications for ambulatory monitoring in angina pectoris. Am J Cardiol 1984; 54:1321-1325.

12. Parker JO, Chiong MA, West RO, Case RB. Sequential alterations in myocardial lactate metabolism, S-T segments, and left ventricular function during pacing induced angina. Circulation 1969; 40:113-131.

13. Johnson SM, Mauritson DR, Winniford MD, Willerson J, Firth B, Cary J, Hillis D. Continuous electrocardiographic monitoring in patients with unstable angina pectoris; identification of high-risk subgroup with severe coronary disease, variant angina, and/or impaired early prognosis. Am Heart J 1982; 103:4-12.

14. Gottlieb SO, Weisfeldt ML, Ouyang P, Mellits D, Gerstenblith G. Silent ischemia as a marker for early unfavorable outcomes in patients with unstable angina. N Engl J Med 1986; 314:12141219.

15. Tzivoni D, Benhorin J, Gavish A, Stern S. Holter recordings during treadmill testing in assessing myocardial ischemic changes. Am J Cardiol 1985; 55:1200-1203.

16. Rose GA, Blackburn H. Cardiovascular Survey Methods, World Health Organization, Genva, 1968.

17. Greenberg HM, Gillespie J, Dwyer EM Jr, The Multicenter Post-Infarction Research Group. A new electrocardiographic classification for post-myocardial infarction clinical trials. Am J Cardiol 1987; 59:1057-1063.

18. Wackers F, Fetterman RC, Mattera JA, Clements JP. Quantitative planar thallium-201 stress scintigraphy: a critical evaluation of the method. J Nuc Med 1985; 15:46-66.

19. Bodenheimer MM, Banka VS, Fooshee C, Hermann GA, Helfant RH. Relationship between regional myocardial perfusion and the presence, severity and reversibility of asynergy in patients with coronary heart disease. Circulation 1978; 5:789.

20. Madeira SW Jr, Bodenheimer MM, Banka VS, Agarwal JB, Weintraub WS, Helfant RH. Quantitative thallium-201 imaging: limitations in detecting pathophysiologically significant obstructive coronary artery disease. Am Heart J 1984; 108:1448-1454.

21. McCarthy DM, Makler PT Jr. Potential limitations of quantitative thallium scanning. Am J Cardiol 1985; 55:215-217.

22. Kaul S, Boucher CA, Newell JB, Chesler DA, Greenberg JM, Okada RD, Strauss HM, Dinsmore RE, Pohost GM. Determination of the quantitative thallium imaging variables that optimize detection of coronary artery disease. J Am Coll Cardiol 1986; 7:527-537.

23. Hinkle L, Thaler HT. Clinical classification of cardiac death. Circulation 1982; 65:457-461.

24. Cox DR. Regression models and life-tables. J Stat Soc (B) 1972; 34:187-220.

25. Fleiss JL. Statistical methods for rates and proportions. 2nd ed. New York, John Wiley, 1981; 138-143.

26. Gibson R, Watson D, Craddock G, Crampton R, Kaiser D, Denny M, Beller G. Prediction of cardiac events aftr uncomplicated myocardial infarction: a prospective study comparing predischarge exercise thallium-201 scintigraphy and coronary angiography. Circulation 1983; 68:321-336.

10

SILENT MYOCARDIAL ISCHEMIA AND SUDDEN CARDIAC DEATH

LEONARD N. HOROWITZ, M.D.

Philadelphia Heart Institute, Presbyterian-University of Pennsylvania Medical Center, Philadelphia, Pennsylvania

ABSTRACT

Coronary artery disease is the major cause of death in Western society and the mechanism of death is usually a malignant ventricular arrhythmia. These arrhythmias commonly cause sudden cardiac death and in fact the initial clinical manifestation of coronary artery disease is sudden cardiac death in a substantial number of patients. These malignant ventricular arrhythmias may result from one or more of several mechanisms. They may be caused by scarring and an electrophysiologic-anatomic melieu which allows the initiation of sustained ventricular arrhythmias or acute myocardial infarction. Recently, interest has been growing in the study of silent myocardial ischemia and its role in sudden cardiac death. This chapter reviews the relationship between silent myocardial ischemia and sudden cardiac death.

INTRODUCTION

Sudden cardiac death is the leading cause of death in middle-aged people in Western civilization. Estimates of the incidence of sudden death in the United States alone reach approximately 450,000 people per year. Moreover, approximately 50% of all deaths from coronary artery disease are sudden and the majority of patients who die suddenly are found to have coronary artery disease. There is no question that the problem of sudden cardiac death and coronary artery disease are intertwined (1-3).

Sudden cardiac death, although variably defined, is generally thought to be instantaneous or occurring over a very short period of time. Although death occurs instantaneously, it usually occurs in the setting of cardiovascular disease and it has generally been thought that prodromal symptoms have been misinterpreted or ignored by victims and even their physicians (3). More problematic is the recognition of patients with coronary artery disease in whom symptoms are absent or the severity of the underlying coronary artery disease is not accurately reflected by the level of symptoms. The concept of silent myocardial ischemia has gained considerable support in the past several years. Asymptomatic myocardial ischemia has been reported in patients with stable angina as well as pre-infarction syndromes and myocardial infarction (4-6). More importantly, the prognosis in patients with silent myocardial ischemia is worse than in comparable patients without this finding (7,8).

SILENT MYOCARDIAL ISCHEMIA AND MALIGNANT VENTRICULAR ARRHYTHMIAS

It is reasonable, therefore, to investigate the relationship between silent myocardial ischemia and the malignant ventricular arrhythmias which produce sudden death. Few opportunities to directly observe the electrocardiographic mechanism of sudden cardiac death limit our ability to directly study this phenomenon; however, increasing examples of fortuitos ambulatory electrocardiographic monitor recordings during episodes of sudden death have allowed us to gain some insight. Most data show that ventricular tachyarrhythmias are infrequently associated with silent myocardial ischemia (9). In most cases of sudden cardiac death in which a Holter monitoring recording is available, the proximate cause of death is a ventricular tachyarrhythmia. Prior to the widespread use of Holter monitoring, it was thought that the majority of patients who suffered sudden cardiac death developed *de novo* ventricular fibrillation (10). However, numerous examples of Holter monitoring recordings have shown that the initial rhythm is usually a rapid ventricular tachycardia which degenerates to ventricular fibrillation (11-14). In most electrocardiographic recordings preceding fatal ventricular tachyarrhythmias, no significant ST segment alterations have been observed.

Thus in a highly selected group of patients, the majority of whom have known heart disease and arrhythmias, the fatal ventricular tachyarrhythmias do not appear to be related to acute myocardial ischemia, silent or painful. It is interesting to note that at least one report of a patient who died suddenly during Holter monitoring in whom heart disease was not previously known showed ST segment elevation immediately prior to fatal ventricular fibrillation (13). Our current understanding of the association between acute ischemia and these lethal arrhythmias may be skewed by the fact that most patients who undergo Holter monitoring have known heart disease, frequently a prior myocardial infarction, and the mechanism of lethal malignant ventricular arrhythmias in this group may be different than those patients in whom the first manifestation of coronary artery disease is sudden death.

SILENT MYOCARDIAL ISCHEMIA AND LETHAL BRADYARRHYTHMIAS

Approximately 20% of cardiac arrests which occurred during Holter monitoring are caused by bradyarrhythmias and asystole (14,15). Based on data obtained from ST segment analysis, it appears that silent ischemia may play a greater role in such sudden deaths than in those due to ventricular tachyarrhythmias.

The bradyarrhythmias associated with sudden cardiac death range from sinus arrest and slow junctional or idioventricular rhythms to high-grade AV block and asystole. Several case reports have identified preceding ST segment deviations which strongly suggested ischemia (14-17).

IS THERE AN ASSOCIATION BETWEEN SILENT MYOCARDIAL ISCHEMIA AND MALIGNANT ARRHYTHMIAS?

One group of patients with reversible myocardial ischemia that has been extensively studied is the group of patients with variant angina pectoris. Prinzmetal and his co-workers described the syndrome of ST segment elevation and ventricular arrhythmias nearly 30 years ago (18) and this was documented to be caused by coronary artery spasm 15 years later (19). The incidence of sudden death in patients with variant angina ranges from 4 to 15% and is usually assumed to be related to arrhythmias produced by acute myocardial ischemia (20,21). In patients with variant angina pectoris, over 1/3 of episodes of ST segment elevation may be asymptomatic and severe arrhythmias may also be noted during such asymptomatic periods of myocardial ischemia. Thus in this special situation, namely variant angina pectoris and coronary artery spasm, silent myocardial ischemia can be associated with arrhythmias, both bradyarrhythmias and tachyarrhythmias, which can produce sudden cardiac death. It must be emphasized that the prevalence of variant angina pectoris is low and that this explains a small percentage of sudden cardiac deaths, but it does provide some insight into the association between acute myocardial ischemia and malignant arrhythmias.

In a more typical population of patients who have survived out-of-hospital cardiac arrest, a high prevalence of reversible myocardial ischemia has been shown. In one study of 21 survivors of out-of-hospital cardiac arrest, thallium scintigraphy showed reversible defects suggestive of ischemia in 77% of patients (20). Interesting, in the majority of these patients angina was not reported during the exercise tolerance test. Sharma and co-workers (23) have also demonstrated that in survivors of out-of-hospital cardiac arrest, painless myocardial ischemia is frequently provoked by exercise. In the latter study, ST segment depression and wall motion abnormalities occurred during exercise without angina. These studies suggest that at least in one population of patients who suffer out-of-hospital cardiac arrest, painless myocardial ischemia may play a role.

Interestingly, patients with recurrent sustained ventricular tachycardia, some of whom may also suffer cardiac arrest with their arrhythmia, have a very low incidence of exercise induced myocardial ischemia (24). While these patients do have large areas of myocardial scar detected by thallium scintigraphy and akinesia or dyskinesia detected by ventriculography, reversible ischemia does not appear to be a prominent part of this clinical syndrome. Thus it may be that these patients represent a different part of the spectrum of patients with cardiac arrest, namely, those with a fixed anatomic-pathologic substrate which does not require acute ischemia for precipitation of the arrhythmia.

CONCLUSION

The association between sudden cardiac death and silent myocardial ischemia continues to evolve. Since both phenomena are prevalent, it would not be surprising that both would occur in the same patient occasionally. We are just emerging from the phenomenologic stage into a period of appropriately designed prospective studies of the relationship between silent myocardial ischemia and malignant arrhythmias. In certain patient groups there does appear to be a relationship. The clinical significance and appropriate management of silent myocardial ischemia in this setting remains to be resolved.

REFERENCES

1. Myerberg, R.J., Conde, C.A., Sung, R.J., Mayorga-Cortes, A., Mallon, S.M., Sheps, D.S., Appel, R.A., Castellanos, A. Clinical electrophysiologic and hemodynamic profile of patients resuscitated from prehospital cardiac arrest. Am. J. Med. 1980;68:568-576.
2. 1987 Heart Facts, American Heart Association.
3. Goldstein, S., Medendorp, S.V., Landis, J.R., Wolfe, R.A., Leighton, R., Ritter, G., Vasu, M., Acheson, A. Analysis of cardiac symptoms preceding cardiac arrest. Am. J. Cardiol. 1986;58:1195-1198.
4. Tzivoni, D., Gavish, A., Benhorin, J., Keren, A., Stern, S. Myocardial ischemia during daily activities and stress. Am. J. Cardiol. 1986;58:47B-50B.

5. Cecchi, A.C., Dorellini, E.V., Morchi, F., Pucci, P., Santoro, G.M., Fazzini, P.F. Silent myocardial ischemia during ambulatory electrocardiographic monitoring in patients with effort angina. J. Am. Coll. Cardiol. 1983;1:934-939.
6. Kannel, W.B., Abbott, R.D. Incidence and prognosis of unrecognized myocardial infarction. An update on the Framingham study. N. Engl. J. Med. 1984;311:1144-1147.
7. Hickman, J.R., Jr., Uhl, G.S., Cook, R.L., Engel, P.J., Hopkirk, A. A natural history study of asymptomatic coronary disease (abstr.) Am. J. Cardiol. 1980;45:422.
8. Langou, R.A., Huang, E.K., Kelley, M.J., Cohen, L.S. Predicted accuracy of coronary artery classification and abnormal exercise test for coronary artery disease in asymptomatic men. Circulation 1980;62:1196-1203.
9. Meissner, M.D., Morganroth, J. Silent myocardial ischemia as a mechanism of sudden cardiac death. In Pepine CJ, ed. Silent Myocardial Ischemia. Philadelphia: WB Saunders, 1986:593-605.
10. Adgey, A.A.J., Scott, M.E., Allen, J.D., Nelson, P.G., Geddes, J.S., Zaidi, S.A., Pantridge, J.F. Management of ventricular fibrillation outside hospital. Lancet 1969;1:1169-1172.
11. Bliefer, S.B., Bleiter, D.J., Hansmann, D.R., Sheppard, J.J., Karpman, H.L. Diagnosis of occult arrhythmias by Holter electrocardiography. Prog. Cardiovasc. Dis. 1974;16:569-599.
12. Gradman, A.H., Bell, P.A., DeBusk, R.F. Sudden death during ambulatory monitoring: clinical and electrocardiographic correlations. Report of a case. Circulation 1977;55:210-211.
13. Savage D.D., Castelli, W.P., Anderson, S.J., Kannel, W.B. Sudden unexpected death during ambulatory electrocardiographic monitoring: the Framingham study. Am. J. Med. 1983;74:148-152.
14. Panidis, I.P., Morganroth, J. Sudden death in hospitalized patients: cardiac rhythm disturbances detected by ambulatory electrocardiographic monitoring. J. Am. Coll. Cardiol. 1983;2:798-805.
15. Clark, M.B., Dwyer, E.M., Greenberg, H. Sudden death during ambulatory monitoring. Analysis of six cases. Am. J. Med. 1983;75:801-806.
16. Salerno, D., Hodges, M., Graham, E., Asinger, R.W., Mikell, F.L. Fatal cardiac arrest during continuous ambulatory monitoring. N. Engl. J. Med. 1981,305:700.

17. Kempf, F.C., Josephson, M.E. Cardiac arrest recorded on ambulatory electrocardiograms. Am. J. Cardiol. 1984;53:1577-1582.
18. Prinzmetal, M., Kennamer, R., Merliss, R., Wada, T., Bor, N. Angina pectoris - I. A variant form of angina pectoris. Am. J. Med. 1959;27:375-388.
19. Oliva, P.B., Potts, D.E., Pluss, R.G. Coronary arterial spasm in Prinzmetal's angina: documentation by coronary arteriography. N. Engl. J. Med. 1973;288:745-751.
20. Maseri, A., Severi, S., DeNes, M., L'Abbate, A., Chierchia, S., Marzilli, M., Ballestra, A.M., Parodi, O., Biagini, A., Distante, A. "Variant" angina. One aspect of a continuous spectrum of vasospastic myocardial ischemia. Am. J. Cardiol. 1978;42:1019-1035.
21. Miller, D.D., Waters, D.D., Szlachcic, J., Theroux, P. Clinical characteristics associated with sudden death in patients with variant angina. Circulation 1982;66:588-592.
22. Ritchie, J.L., Hamilton, G.W., Trobaugh, G.B., Weaver, W.D., Williams, D.L., Cobb, L.A. Myocardial imaging and radionulcide angiography in survivors of sudden cardiac death due to ventricular fibrillation: preliminary report. Am. J. Cardiol. 1977;39:852-857.
23. Sharma, B., Asinger, R., Francis, G.S., Hodges, M., Wyeth, R.P. Demonstration of exercise-induced painless myocardial ischemia in survivors of out-of-hospital ventricular fibrillation. Am. J. Cardiol. 1987;59:740-745.
24. Sellers, T.D., Beller, G.A., Gibson, R.S., Watson, D.D., DiMarco, J.P. Prevalence of ischemia by quantitative thallium-201 scintigraphy in patients with ventricular tachycardia or fibrillation inducible by programmed stimulation. Am. J. Cardiol. 1987;59:828-832.

DISCUSSION - 3

Dr. Morganroth: In Missme what thoughts have you given to the confounding influence of the various therapies that these patients will be put on or changed to or from during the course of the trial.

Dr. Bigger: We gave a lot of consideration to that question. In fact we debated for about 6 months in the planning phase about whether or not to take them off therapy to evaluate ischemia. We decided that was not what we wanted to do. It would depend on the objectives what you decided to do, but our major objective was to see if patients that were stable, at least were considered stable by their physician after having had two to four to six months to stabilize the patient after a major event that caused hospitalization in an intensive or a step-down kind of care unit, whether or not the ST depression in that situation were related to outcomes. It seemed wrong to us at a multicenter study to do something that might have some hazard, taking people off medication and then to assess their ischemic risk if you would or their ischemic situation off medication and put them right back on and follow them didn't seem that logical to us either. The other side of your question which may be more what you are asking is how are we going to deal with the confounding due to treatment? The main effects we would estimate that it showed in the absence of consideration of treatment and then we would add treatment into the model and see how much effect attributable to the ST segment question was accounted for by treatment. It is the standard. It is the best that can be done. It is never as nice as having like randomized assignment to the drugs.

Dr. Morganroth: What percent of 1000 patients will not be on beta blockers, calcium blockers, or nitrates?

Dr. Bigger: We did a survey of the hospitals that are involved and based on that, and I don't see anything new that would encourage people to increase the use of nitrates, calcium channel blockers or beta blockers on the horizon. If anything there may be some discouraging news coming along in the near future. About 40% are on beta blockers, 40% on calcium channel blockers and about 43-50% on nitrates and 25% are on two or more treatments combined. Everybody that has angina is going to be on anti-anginal medication or maybe even anti-ischemic medications and the ones post-infarction who do not have any angina, it is interesting that a third of the people post-infarction will have what is called by a doctor anyway, angina before they go home and before the first year ends, half the patients have had that label attached to them at one time or another.

Dr. Lipicky: What thinking process led to describing the natural history as opposed to an intervention?

Dr. Bigger: We were interested particularly in the episodes of ST depression, the 10 to 20 minute episodes that you see in Holter recordings. We have done some preliminary recordings post-infarction and we found that about a third of the patients have these say 3 months after discharge from the hospital. It is about that and Dan Savoni in our group did a study about the same size as ours but 100 patients. He also found about that prevalence in several other smaller studies found the same thing. So I think that is about right, and we don't know that much about their significance in that setting. There are a lot of confounding variables that Hal Kennedy mentioned that could give you ST deviations and not represent ischemia and so forth. We didn't think we knew enough about it at the present time to plan an intervention trial and we just didn't think it was well enough characterized. If you had a strong hypothesis and you were coming off a base of say an industrial perspective and a product that you had a lot of confidence in, you might say, we'll do a big trial and we'll learn about natural history in the placebo group or something of that sort. We thought we needed not only natural history but probably more feasibility information before doing trials that use mortality or mortality plus infarction that has relatively rare events as end points which means large numbers of patients. So we just didn't think we were prepared to do it. Maybe some other group would have the insight to do that.

Dr. Lipicky: How clinically different do you think the population that you will be studying is from the populations that we were shown earlier today in terms of events associated with silent ischemia?

Dr. Bigger: I really don't know. It is not well explored at the present time. This is a sort of a bursting scene and I am talking now not about the exercise information which I think is a little better developed. But I think for a Holter event that we are talking about, primarily the studies have been done to gain confidence into the fact that there was a real finding. Maybe in the last 18-20 months, maybe two years, people have been gaining more confidence and turning to other questions, but primarily they are people who have had angina pectoris and also had a positive exercise test, and then had Holter studies and all of them had exercise ischemia and all of them had angina pectoris. The fact was many of these episodes on Holter weren't associated with pain only about 20% were. I just don't think we have a lot of association with end points like reinfarction and death at the present time and there are many populations that haven't even been looked at as of yet.

Dr. Temple: This is question for you Joel. The BHAT data base includes a lot of Holters and the question I have is whether those can be analyzed after the fact for ischemic events, and whether that would allow you to say something about whether the benefits of beta blocker therapy were found only in certain subsets or whether there is any predictive value in the placebo groups or anything. Is that data retrievable and useable for that purpose?

Dr. Morganroth: The answer is yes. In fact the tapes are being looked at to specifically select a subset of patients who were randomized to placebo versus those who were randomized to propranolol. We'll look at mortality end points and the ST segment changes that occurred in each group relative to therapy. How good the quality of those tapes are from a technical point of view and how well the ST's can be read with current equipment using tapes which were recorded several years ago, we'll find out.

Dr. Temple: Do you recall the specific analysis that was done on effect in people as determined by whether they did or did not have angina persisting after treatment. The trial included both, although you couldn't be in it if you had to be on a beta blocker so that probably excluded a number of angina patients.

Dr. Morganroth: Angina was one of the secondary end points that we looked at so that kind of data was recorded in a follow-up period. Thus that will be one of the potential end points one could use in this study in addition to mortality.

Dr. Temple: Tom, is one of your thoughts that there is a characteristic prolonged ischemic episode that occurs in some people and not in others and that that may have something to do with outcome and perhaps something to do with what drug you are on?

Dr. Bigger: I think we are worried about how widely applicable this is. Certainly a lot of problems with angina patients who haven't had previous infarction and aren't on a lot of medications aside from their anti-anginal or anti-ischemic medication. The electrocardiograms at baseline or between events are pretty clean. The t-wave is O.K., ST segments aren't abbreviated.
Post-infarction is a harder thing. You are more likely to have t waves turned over, persistent ST segment changes, bundle branch blocks and a lot of other things that are going to give Holters a lot of problems. But looking at the data in the angina population where you see the ST segments come down and look horizontal and very typical of ischemia as we have learned to recognize them from analyzing exercise ECG's and stay down for a typical episode median about 12, 10-20 minutes, is sort of where most of them are, and it is usually not that common. It has about the same prevalence as unsustained VT in a post-infarction population. It is about twice that prevalent and it is usually one or two episodes a day, something of that sort in patients who have it. It is not that common, but total time usually adds up in persons that have it, ranges around 20-60 minutes and I think everyone is concerned, very concerned, when you think about that period of ischemia going on every day and assumes that it may have some prognostic significance.

Dr. Temple: So if you were to find that these had prognostic significance, you would then consider a trial in which some series of maneuvers to try to eliminate them were compared with other maneuvers.

Dr. Bigger: That would be the logical thing to do. I don't know. Things are moving very fast and the window may close before it is possible to get that kind of information. In fact I am very pleased that we are going to be collecting information for a relatively short period of time because I think even in natural history studies the window could close pretty soon. Is anyone thinking about doing either intervention trials placebo controlled or natural history studies I think ought to get moving because the window is closing.

Dr. Weiner: I just have one comment. I understand your problem about trying to stabilize patients but I would suggest that by waiting 2-6 months after acute myocardial infarction or unstable angina, you are going to essentially weed out the more high risk patients and your population is going to resemble the CASS population. The events rate in the CASS population was pretty low in medically treated patients followed over the years, so I would have to predict that your event rate would be fairly small in your population by waiting rather than try to undergo some studies earlier, but I can understand your reason for trying to stabilize.

Dr. Bigger: We don't want so many drop outs that we can't characterize the population. I take your point. We are estimating a 13% 2-year event rate and we are not using just cardiac death, but cardiac death plus non-fatal reinfarction plus hospitalized unstable angina. I think you are right. We thought about it and we thought we might just destroy the trial in attempting to take unstable patients in and having them dropping out due to coronary artery bypass surgery, angioplasty and other things doctors make decisions about and we wanted to avoid having a huge number of drop outs for conventional treatments. I don't know anyway out of it. I take your point.

Dr. Morganroth: Of the 500,000 sudden cardiac deaths out of hospital per year, Peter Cohn told us this morning that a good proportion of them, maybe a third, sometimes a half will have had no clinical cardiac event prior to their sudden cardiac death and sudden cardiac death becomes their manifestation of underlying coronary disease. Therefore, it is tempting to suggest a relationship of sudden death to silent myocardial ischemia. We have previously shown on Holter monitoring studies no changes that are at least very obvious in the ST segment in the preceding few beats or minutes before that sudden cardiac death VT-VF episode. This is the mechanism in 80% of cases. The question I have, is how does one put together with the question of silent myocardial ischemia being part of this mechanism that sets off these sudden deaths?

Dr. Horowitz: One of the problems is that if you look at all the published examples of Holters recorded during sudden death, they are obviously all recordings by serendipity. Most of those patients were either being evaluated for or under treatment for arrhythmias. That is not the group that is otherwise healthy and then suddenly drops dead so there is a selection bias in that we get Holters in patients who have manifest heart disease and very often they manifest arrhythmia. We don't often get Holter monitors in people we think are perfectly healthy, so that there is a problem with looking at the anecdotes. By far and away the vast majority of the published examples show ST segment elevation rather than depression when there is an ST segment deviation associated with malignant arrhythmias. There are certainly examples and I showed one of ST segment depression, but there are far more, there are probably 5 ST segment elevation examples for every ST segment depression for example with the exception of the bradyarrhythmias. That is one problem. The patients are known to be ill and that is why the Holter monitoring has generally been gotten. So there is a problem with using the Holter and trying to extrapolate that to the 500,000 deaths a year. The other problem is that there is some suggestion in the literature and my own clinical impression that patients who have sudden death because they have an electrophysiologic problem may be more readily resuscitated than patients who have primarily an ischemic event and that may be part of the reason why the patients with the bradyarrhythmias are not resuscitated very frequently because they are frequently related to ischemia. It may be that we see primarily patients that have mostly an arrhythmic event rather than an ischemic event although that is all supposition. There are a number of problems with looking at the patients who have survived cardiac arrest at this point.

Dr. Cohn: First of all I think that we don't necessarily have to expect to see a 1:1 relation between an ischemic event and VF. We know for example every time a patient has angina, they don't go into VF, yet we know that if we took a patient population with angina, we are going to have a certain percentage of arrhythmic deaths in that population and I think the same analogy has to be made to silent ischemia in totally healthy people. It is this substrate who have repeated ischemic events are going to be the ones to go on to have these electrophysiologic deaths, even though at the time of their death they may not have what we can identify as an ischemic event triggering it off.

Dr. Morganroth: That may mean that getting rid of their silent ischemia may not prevent their sudden death.

Dr. Cohn: That is right. This is something we don't know and it might not prevent them from having an MI again. On the other hand it might. We don't know the answer. Just because we can't make the 1:1 correlation, I think that is the important thing. Looking backwards, it is obvious that as was mentioned earlier today, over and over again, the individuals at risk for cardiac mortality as you have heard over and over are those that have ischemic events, advanced disease, some amount of LV dysfunction. We all agree on that. I think whether or not they have pain or not is really irrelevant. They are the ones at high risk and the trials that you have talked about and we have talked about will attempt to answer the question of whether or not we can influence mortality or not. Whether or not this should be the end point for an FDA approval, is another argument entirely. To me this is the only situation we know where we have to prove a mortality change to get an indication to use a drug.

IV. THERAPY AND FDA CLAIMS

11

ANTIANGINAL DRUG THERAPY FOR SILENT MYOCARDIAL ISCHEMIA: ADRENERGIC BLOCKERS AND CALCIUM ENTRY BLOCKERS

William H. Frishman M.D.

Beta-adrenergic blocking drugs (1), alpha-beta-adrenergic blocking drugs (2), and calcium antagonists (3,4), used alone and in combination, have been shown to be effective in the therapy of symptomatic ischemic heart disease by relieving angina pectoris and reducing the intensity of associated myocardial ischemia.

Recently, close attention has been given to the problem of silent ischemia, or ischemia without symptoms. This condition was recognized over a half century ago when some asymptomatic patients were shown to have reversible ECG changes suggestive of myocardial ischemia during the Master's two-step exam. Recently, technology has been developed to identify asymptomatic transient ischemic episodes using the ambulatory ECG (5,6). Positron emission imaging techniques have validated that these silent ischemic episodes are indicative of true myocardial ischemia (7). The pioneering contributions of Cohn, Maseri, Pepine, Deanfield, Selwyn, and their associates have clearly demonstrated the frequent occurrence of silent ischemic episodes in patients with symptomatic angina and coronary artery disease documented by angiography (8-11). Gottlieb and Gerstenblith have demonstrated the unfavorable prognosis of continued silent ischemia in patients with unstable angina (12). Thus, all antianginal therapies must also be shown to be anti-ischemic if the problem of silent ischemia is to be dealt with in a satisfactory manner.

There are multiple studies available now that have shown favorable effects of beta-adrenergic blockers (13,14), alpha-beta-adrenergic blockers (15), and calcium antagonists on episodes of asymptomatic transient myocardial ischemia observed by ambulatory ECG monitoring in patients with angina and/or coronary artery disease (11). In this chapter, the clinical experiences with these drugs in silent myocardial ischemia will be reviewed.

ADRENERGIC BLOCKERS

Alpha-Adrenergic Blockers

Although alpha-blockers are vasodilators, their clinical utility in symptomatic ischemia is not yet defined (16). There are no reports yet describing effects of alpha-adrenergic blockers on silent myocardial ischemia.

Beta-Adrenergic Blockers

Beta-adrenergic blockers have been a clinical mainstay of long-term antianginal therapy for over 20 years (1). Beneficial effects on stable angina are well known, but some controversy was raised regarding their utility as monotherapy in vasospastic angina syndromes (17). Certainly, in combination with nitrates and calcium antagonists, their usefulness in all forms of angina has been proven beyond question (1).

As will be discussed later in the section on calcium antagonists, propranolol as monotherapy has been shown to be as effective as verapamil and nifedipine in reducing both painful and silent ischemic episodes (evidenced on the ambulatory ECG) in patients with angina pectoris. When combined with nifedipine, the combination appears more effective than with either drug alone.

Seventy-three patients, aged 41-75 years, with established stable exertional angina pectoris, were studied by Khurmi et al (18) in a double-blind fashion, to confirm the efficacy of 80 mg propranolol administered three times daily, and to examine its effects on ST segment changes in the electrocardiogram by ambulatory ST segment monitoring and exercise testing, using on-line computer analysis. During ambulatory monitoring, episodes of ST segment depression were significantly reduced by propranolol compared with placebo treatment. The total duration of ST segment depression was also significantly reduced by active treatment and the maximal depth of ST segment depression was reduced. Exercise time was improved by propranolol. The authors concluded that propranolol was an effective antianginal agent which also improves the ST segment changes during controlled, as well as uncontrolled conditions, related to the drug's ability to lower the heart rate and rate-pressure product.

Gottlieb et al evaluated 81 patients with unstable angina treated with maximal nitrate and calcium-channel blocker (nifedipine) therapy, where propranolol or placebo was added as additional treatment (19). There was a greater reduction in symptomatic episodes of angina and nitroglycerin consumption with propranolol. Continuous ECG recordings for ischemic ST segment changes revealed fewer daily ischemic episodes (painful or silent) in the propranolol group than in the placebo group, and a shorter duration of ischemia. The authors concluded that the addition of propranolol in patients with unstable angina receiving nitrates and nifedipine reduces the frequency and duration of symptomatic and silent ischemic episodes.

Cohn et al (20) studied the effects of propranolol in 11 patients with coronary artery disease and ECG evidence of silent myocardial ischemia on exercise testing. Using gated radionuclide imaging of the left ventricle, they demonstrated improved global ventricular functioning with beta-blocker therapy (propranolol, timolol) compared to baseline. They concluded that beta-adrenergic blockade can effectively improve the abnormalities in exercise left ventricular function in patients with coronary artery disease and silent myocardial ischemia.

Quyyumi and his associates compared the antianginal effects of atenolol and pindolol in patients with effort angina and nocturnal angina (21). Pindolol 5 mg three times daily and atenolol 100 mg daily were given for five days each in a double-blind, randomized manner. Daytime and nocturnal resting heart rates and the frequency of angina were significantly reduced by atenolol compared to pindolol. The duration of exercise was significantly increased and the frequency, duration and magnitude of daytime and nocturnal episodes of ST segment depression on ambulatory ECG monitoring were reduced by atenolol. They concluded that resting heart rate reduction is important in the treatment of effort and nocturnal angina, and that partial agonist activity in a beta-blocker may not be a desirable property.

Alpha-Beta-Adrenergic Blockade

Labetalol, the first alpha-beta-adrenergic blocker marketed in the world, has been shown to be effective in the treatment of hypertensive patients with angina pectoris, by lowering blood pressure and reducing anginal episodes (22). Quyyumi and his associates compared placebo to labetalol in patients with chronic stable angina pectoris (23). They observed that compared to placebo, labetalol reduced the frequency of angina and exercise tolerance was prolonged. The drug reduced heart rate and the frequency and duration of ST segment depressions on ambulatory monitoring by 56% and 73% respectively, compared to placebo.

Conclusion

Most beta-adrenergic blockers and the alpha-beta-blocker labetalol appear to be effective in reducing both painful and silent ischemic episodes, when used alone or in combination with other antianginal drugs.

CALCIUM ANTAGONISTS

Verapamil

Verapamil is a calcium antagonist similar in structure to papaverine. It has vasodilator and electrophysiologic activities which have allowed the drug to be used in patients with supraventricular arrhythmias, stable and unstable angina, and systemic hypertension (3).

Johnson et al studied 16 patients with documented variant angina (Prinzmetal type) in a placebo-controlled study of verapamil (24). This study was complicated by the fact that patients were on concomitant therapy which included isosorbide dinitrate and digoxin. Patients were randomized to receive either verapamil or placebo for four months after a one month placebo run-in period. The patients were then crossed over to receive the other regimen for an additional four months. Episodes of angina, nitroglycerin consumption, and transient ST-segment shifts detected on a weekly ambulatory ECG exam were assessed. Episodes of angina/week, nitroglycerin consumed/week were reduced, as well as transient ischemic ECG changes, many of which were unassociated with pain.

The same group of investigators compared the effects of nifedipine to verapamil in a similar group of patients with variant angina (25). This was not a direct comparison though, since verapamil was administered as part of a blinded, placebo-controlled study, whereas nifedipine was administered in open-label fashion to patients who had already completed the blinded trial. In comparing the effects of the two drugs, both drugs appeared equally effective in reducing angina attacks, nitroglycerin consumption, and transient ischemic episodes observed on a weekly ambulatory ECG exam.

In a study of patients with unstable vasospastic angina at rest who were studied in a hospital setting, verapamil but not propranolol significantly reduced the number of symptomatic and asymptomatic episodes of transient ischemia detected by continuous ECG monitoring (26). These investigators concluded that verapamil was more effective than propranolol in patients with unstable angina.

Bala Subramanian and his associates examined 22 patients with stable angina pectoris, comparing propranolol 240 mg/day to verapamil 360 mg/day in a double-blind, placebo-controlled trial (27). Patients were only receiving the study drugs. Although these investigators found verapamil to prolong exercise time more effectively than propranolol, they could discern no differences between the drugs in their favorable effects on transient ischemia detected on an ambulatory ECG.

These same investigators compared nifedipine (30 mg/day) to verapamil (360 mg/day) in 28 patients with chronic stable angina, using a similar protocol (28). Overall, they showed verapamil to be more effective than nifedipine in prolonging exercise time. However, unlike the previous study comparing propranolol to verapamil, they demonstrated that verapamil was more effective than nifedipine in reducing ischemic episodes on the ambulatory ECG. They also noted that some patients demonstrated increased ischemic episodes with nifedipine. The investigators proposed that the different effects of nifedipine and verapamil on episodes of ambulatory ST-segment depression were related to the different effects the two drugs have on heart rate (28).

In conclusion, all the published data would suggest that verapamil is an effective drug for reducing painful and silent episodes of transient ischemia in patients with variant angina (Prinzmetal type), unstable angina, and stable angina.

Nifedipine

Nifedipine is a dihydropyridine compound which is a calcium antagonist similar in structure to the newer calcium antagonists (nitrendipine, nicardipine, nimodipine, nivaldipine, amlodipine, etc.). It is an extremely potent coronary and systemic vasodilator which is clinically useful in patients with hypertension and/or angina pectoris. It has a different hemodynamic profile than verapamil, which relates to the increased sympathetic nervous system activity observed after nifedipine administration which is not seen with verapamil (3). Nifedipine has been studied in patients with episodes of silent ischemia with, conflicting reports regarding the drug's efficacy in the literature.

As mentioned earlier, investigators in an uncontrolled study of patients with variant angina have shown a favorable effect of nifedipine on episodes of symptomatic and asymptomatic myocardial ischemia detected by continuous ambulatory ECG monitoring (25).

Oakley et al (29) treated six men with severe angina with propranolol or nifedipine, and propranolol plus nifedipine, while episodes of both painful and silent ECG ST-segment depressions were recorded by ambulatory monitoring. All three treatment regimens reduced the total number of ischemic episodes, both painful and silent, but the combination of propranolol plus nifedipine was significantly superior to either drug alone.

Dargie and his associates (30) also evaluated the actions of nifedipine and propranolol and their combination in patients with stable angina pectoris. They utilized doses of nifedipine of 30 and 60 mg/day and propranolol 240 and 480 mg/day, administered in three divided doses as monotherapies, and in combination. The investigators observed that both drugs in the doses administered improved exercise tolerance, reduced angina attack frequency, and reduced nitroglycerin consumption. Combination therapy was only slightly better than monotherapy. Sixty percent of the ischemic episodes detected by ambulatory ECG monitoring in this study were silent. Both propranolol and nifedipine monotherapies reduced episodes of ST-segment depression, both painful and silent, in a similar fashion. Combination therapy was slightly better than either monotherapy.

Cocco and co-workers (31), in a single-blind, randomized, parallel design study of patients with stable angina undergoing ambulatory ECG monitoring, found 12 patients with silent ischemic episodes at rest. In six of seven patients, silent ischemia was reduced or eliminated while patients were taking nifedipine. In contrast, only one of five patients showed improvement while taking pindolol.

In contrast to the studies showing favorable effects of nifedipine on silent myocardial ischemia, Bala Subramanian et al (28), as noted above, could find no favorable effect on this parameter using similar doses of nifedipine in patients with stable angina. Similar technologies were utilized to assess transient myocardial ischemia in these studies, and heart rates on nifedipine therapy were similar. The explanation for this difference is not yet apparent.

In conclusion, nifedipine appears to be effective when used alone or in combination with beta-blockers for silent myocardial ischemia; however, this observation has not been a universal one and more clinical studies with the drug are necessary.

Diltiazem

Diltiazem is a benzothiazepine compound that is structurally unrelated to other vasodilators. It has different hemodynamic actions than nifedipine and different electrophysiologic actions than nifedipine and verapamil (3). The drug is clinically useful in patients with angina and/or hypertension, and appears to be useful in reducing morbidity and mortality in patients who survived subendocardial wall myocardial infarction.

There is a paucity of data regarding the effects of diltiazem on silent myocardial ischemia. Frishman and his colleagues (32) studied the effects of diltiazem on the ambulatory ECG designed for ST-segment analysis. In this placebo-controlled, double-blind study of 20 patients with chronic stable angina, diltiazem 360 mg/day was found to reduce episodes of angina and nitroglycerin consumption, while improving exercise tolerance, when compared to placebo therapy. Diltiazem was found to reduce the number of episodes of silent ischemia detected over a 24 hour period. The drug also reduced the length of the individual episodes. Combination therapy with nifedipine provided no further advantage. With abrupt withdrawal of active therapy, patients returned to their pretreatment states with no evidence of an overshoot.

In conclusion, diltiazem appears to be effective in the treatment of silent and painful ischemic episodes in patients with chronic stable angina. There is no information yet available regarding the effects of diltiazem on silent ischemic episodes in patients with variant and unstable angina syndromes.

COMBINATION DRUG THERAPY

As described throughout this chapter, antianginal drugs used in combination may provide greater efficacy in treating painful and silent ischemic episodes than with monotherapy. More work needs to be done, however, comparing different combination regimens for treatment of myocardial ischemia.

ANTI-PLATELET DRUGS

Anti-platelet drugs have been suggested for treatment of ischemia since platelet activation may be playing an important role in various forms of angina (32).

Aspirin

Aspirin is now approved for the treatment of

unstable angina and for prolonging life in survivors of acute myocardial infarction (33). Cherchia et al (34) examined the effects of intravenous aspirin in patients with vasospastic angina, and concluded that the drug was not effective in preventing myocardial ischemia, including painless episodes. In the study using ambulatory ECG recordings, they observed 129 ischemic episodes before aspirin (26 with pain and 103 without pain) and 146 episodes after aspirin (32 with pain and 114 without pain). Similarly, the duration of ischemic episodes did not change with administration of aspirin. The aspirin dose reduced thromboxane $beta_2$ levels to 3% of control levels. Repeated ambulatory monitoring during treatment with combined high-dose nitrates and calcium antagonists showed that the number of ischemic episodes were reduced to less than 20% of those recorded during aspirin administration.

DISCUSSION

Many of the available beta-adrenergic blockers and calcium antagonists appear to be useful in patients with painful and silent ischemic episodes detected on the ECG. More controlled studies need to be done using standardized methodologies for assessing silent myocardial ischemia, to evaluate and compare the different antianginal medications. It is fortunate, however, that the beta-blockers and calcium antagonists, used alone and in combination, appear to not only have favorable effects on painful ischemic episodes, but also on those ischemic episodes not associated with pain.

REFERENCES

1. Frishman, W.H. In: Therapy of Angina Pectoris (Weiner, D., Frishman, W.H., eds), Marcel Dekker Inc., New York, 1986, 83-144.
2. Jee, L.D. and Opie, L.H. Am. J. Cardiol 56: 551-54, 1985.
3. Weiner, D. In: Therapy of Angina Pectoris (Weiner, D., Frishman WH, eds), Marcel Dekker Inc., New York, 1986, 145-204.
4. Frishman, W.H. and Teicher, M. Am. Heart J. 114: 140-47, 1987.
5. Deanfield, J.E., Shea, M., Ribiero, P. et al. Am. J Cardiol. 54: 1195-2000, 1984.
6. Kawanishi, D.T. and Rahimtoola, S.H. Curr. Probl. Cardiol. 12: 509-65, 1987.
7. Deanfield, J.E., Shea, M.J. and Selwyn, A.P. Am. J Med. 79 (Suppl 3A): 18-24, 1985.
8. Cohn, P.F. Am. J Med. 80 (Suppl 4C): 3-8, 1986.
9. Maseri, A., Chierchia ,S., Davies, G., and Glazier, J. Am. J Med. 79 (Suppl 3A): 7-11, 1985.
10. Schang, S.J. and Pepine, C.J. Am. J Cardiol. 39: 396-402, 1977.
11. Pepine, C.J. Am. J Med. 80 (Suppl 4C): 25-34, 1986.
12. Gottlieb, S.O., Weisfeldt, M.L., Ouyang, P., Mellits, E.D. and Gerstenblith, G. N Engl. J Med. 314: 1214-19, 1986.
13. Pepine, C.J., Feldman, R.L., Ludbrook, P., Holland, P., Lambert, C.R., Conti, C.R. and McGrath, P.D. Am. J Cardiol. 58: 38B-42B, 1986.
14. Shell, W.E. Am. J Cardiol. 56: 23I-27I, 1985.
15. Shell, W.E., Kivowitz, C.F., Rubins, S.B. and See, J. Am. Heart J 112: 222-29, 1986.
16. Frishman, W.H. In: Cardiovascular Drug Therapy. Yearbook Publishers, Chicago, 1986; 137-152.
17. Frishman, W.H. Circulation 67: I11-I18, 1983.
18. Khurmi, N.S., Bowles, M.J., O'Hara, M.J. and Raftery, E.B. Clin. Cardiol. 9: 391-97, 1986.
19. Gottlieb, S.O., Weisfeldt, M.L., Ouyang, P., et al. Circulation 73: 331-337, 1986.
20. Cohn, P.F., Brown, E.J., Swinford, R. and Atkins, H. Am. J Cardiol. 57: 521-526, 1986.
21. Quyyumi, A.A., Wright, C., Mockusm L., et al. Br. Med. J 289: 951-53, 1984.

22. Frishman, W.H., Strom, J.A., Kirschner, M., et al. Am. J Cardiol. 48: 917-928, 1981.
23. Quyyumi, A.A., Wright, C., Mockus, et al. Br. Heart J 53: 47-52, 1985.
24. Johnson, S.M., Mauritson, D.R., Willerson, J.T. and Hillis, L.D. N Engl. J Med. 304: 862-66, 1981.
25. Winniford, M.D., Johnson, S.J., Mauritson, D.R., et al. Am. J Cardiol. 50: 913-18, 1982.
26. Parodi, O., Simonetti, I., L'Abbate, A., et al. Am. J Cardiol. 50: 923-28, 1982.
27. Bala Subramanian, V., Bowles, M.J., Davies, A., and Raftery, E. Am. J Cardiol. 50: 1158-63, 1982.
28. Bala Subramanian, V., Bowlesm M.J., Khurmi, N.S., Davies, A.B. and Raftery, E.B. Am. J Cardiol. 50: 1173-79, 1982.
29. Oakley, G.D.G., Fox, K.M., Dargie, H.J. and Selwyn, A,P. Br. Med. J 289: 1540, 1979.
30. Dargie, H.J., Lynch, P.G., Krikler, D.M., Harris, L. and Krikler, S. Am. J Med. 71: 676-82, 1981.
31. Cocco, G., Strozzi, C., Chu, D., et al. Europ. J Cardiol. 10: 59-69, 1979.
32. Frishman, W., Charlap, S., Kimmel, B., Teicher, M. and Strom, J. Clin. Res. 34: 398A, 1986 (abstr).
33. Frishman, W.H. and Miller, K.P. Curr. Prob. Cardiol. 11: 71-136, 1986.
34. Cherchia, S., DeCaterina, R., Cream F., et al. Circulation 66: 702-705, 1982.

22. Friedman, W.F., Strom, J.A., Fleischer, M., et al. [illegible] Cardiol [illegible] 1983.
23. [illegible] 1983.
24. Johnson, R.M., [illegible], Middleton, [illegible] and [illegible] Engl J Med [illegible] 1981.
25. [illegible], Johnson, [illegible] et al. Am J Cardiol [illegible] 1982.
26. [illegible] 1981.
27. [illegible] Am J Cardiol [illegible] 1981.
28. [illegible] Am J Cardiol [illegible] 1983.
29. [illegible] 1979.
30. Parrish, [illegible] Merrick, [illegible] 1982.
31. [illegible] Burgo, [illegible] 1979.
32. Friedman, [illegible] 34: 368A, 1986 (abstract).
33. Friedman, W.F. and [illegible] 1986.
34. [illegible]

12

Therapy For Silent Ischemia: Nitrates

Stephen Scheidt, M.D.
Professor of Clinical Medicine, The New York Hospital-Cornell Medical Center

Nitrates are the oldest of the standard therapeutic agents for ischemic heart disease, first employed as amyl nitrite as reported by Brunton in 1867 (1), and then as nitroglycerin itself by Murrell in 1879 (2). The historical background of nitrate therapy, and particularly its use as a homeopathic remedy, has been elegantly summarized by Fye (3) in a recent review. In spite of long use and unquestioned efficacy in the vast majority of patients with angina, the physiologic actions of nitrates are multiple and complex, with remarkable gaps in our understanding of how efficacy is exerted.

Major hemodynamic actions of nitroglycerin include: 1) profound and rapid venodilation, reducing venous return to the heart and thus preload; 2) systemic arterial and arteriolar dilation, reducing systemic vascular resistance and thus afterload. The combined effects of reducing preload and afterload cause a reduction in left ventricular volume, a decrease in wall tension, and thus a decline in myocardial oxygen consumption. With the reduction in afterload, cardiac index often rises, and so blood pressure falls only modestly in the vast majority of patients; 3) Coronary vasodilation, including dilation of large (conduit) epicardial coronary vessels, dilation of coronary collaterals, prevention or reversal of vasospasm, redistribution of flow toward the more vulnerable subendocardial myocardium, and dilation of stenotic segments. These last 3 attributes distinguish nitroglycerin from other "coronary vasodilators"; for example, dipyridamole and nitroprusside have coronary vasodilating action, but do not appear to enhance coronary collateral flow nor to improve subendocardial flow distribution. As to dilation of stenotic segments of coronary arteries, Brown et al (4) have employed quantitative coronary angiography to demonstrate that substantial increases in luminal cross-sectional area <u>at the site of atherosclerotic narrowing</u> can be produced with administration of nitroglycerin. The anatomic explanation of how a chronic atherosclerotic stenosis might dilate has been provided by Freudenberg and Lichtlen (5). In a study of coronary stenoses, these investigators found that significant portions of the coronary circumference were uninvolved with atheromatous disease in 74% of all stenoses studied.

So long as some portion of the arterial wall is capable of vasomotion (16% of circumference in Freudenberg and Lichtlen's study), and considering the dictates of Poiseuille's Equation (flow varies as the 4th power of the radius), minor degrees of vasoconstriction or vasodilation at the critical point of stenosis should have substantial effects, negative or positive, on coronary flow. Vasodilation with substantial increases in the cross sectional area at the point of maximum stenosis as measured by quantitative coronary angiography has been demonstrated for nitroglycerin and calcium blockers (4).

Clinical Results Using Nitrates for Silent Ischemia

Schang and Pepine first reported using nitrates for silent ischemia in 5 patients treated with hourly sublingual nitroglycerin (6). There was significant reduction in silent ischemic episodes with nitroglycerin as compared to placebo.

In a study of hospitalized patients with vasospastic angina, Distante and co-workers reported major reductions in angina as well as silent ischemic episodes during crossover periods of intravenous isosorbide dinitrate therapy as compared to placebo (7).

Shell (8) has published results in 8 patients in an uncontrolled open label trial of transdermal nitroglycerin for silent ischemia. With transdermal nitroglycerin, titrated to abolish symptomatic events to a mean dose of 10.4 mg/24 hrs., ischemic episodes were reduced from an average of 5.3 ± 3.3 to 0.8 ± 1.2 events per day, while total ischemic time fell from 95.8 ± 87 to 17 ± 27.1 minutes per 24 hours. A randomized double blind parallel trial of transdermal nitroglycerin is currently in progress in Shell's laboratory. Patients have angina and at least three ischemic episodes daily on ambulatory monitoring (using the standard criteria of at least 1 minute of ≥ 1 mm ST-segment depression or elevation). All patients receive beta-blockers, titrated so that resting heart rate is between 60 and 70 beats per minute. The study consists of two weeks each of placebo run-in, 20 mg, 40 mg, and 60 mg of transdermal nitroglycerin applied continuously over a 24 hour period. In preliminary data from the fi¿st 17 patients entered into this trial (9 given placebo run-in and then inactive placebo patches, 8 given placebo run-in and then active transdermal nitroglycerin) the number of episodes of ischemia per 24 hours was unchanged at 8.7 during placebo run-in and 8.2 during the 20 mg placebo phase, whereas the parallel group showed a highly significant decline from 12.1 episodes during placebo run-in to 3.9 episodes with transdermal nitroglycerin 20 mg/24 hours. In the placebo group, total ischemic time per 24 hours was 127 minutes during run-in, unchanged at 115 minutes during 20 mg placebo, as opposed to the active treatment group which showed a significant fall from 121 minutes during run-in to 49 minutes during transdermal nitroglycerin 20 mg/24 hours (p=0.04) (personal communication, W. Shell).

A second ongoing trial from the same laboratory (personal communication, W. Shell) is comparing transdermal nitroglycerin and oral nifedipine for silent ischemia. In this double-blind double-dummy placebo-controlled trial, similar patient selection criteria are utilized, but patients receive no beta blockers or other anti-ischemic therapy. The protocol consists of successive 14 day periods of placebo run-in; placebo; treatment, either transdermal nitroglycerin 15 mg/24 hours or nifedipine 10 mgs orally thrice daily; placebo; the alternate therapy not received during the first active treatment period; and a final placebo period. Exercise stress tests and 24 hour ambulatory monitoring are done on day 13 of each 14 day period. In 8 patients with data analyzed at the time of submission of this manuscript, exercise time did not change with nitroglycerin, and increased 28% with nifedipine. Total ischemic time, though, declined 35% with nifedipine, but 65% with transdermal nitroglycerin (no significance tests done to date due to the small size of the patient group). These preliminary data raise the possibility that nitroglycerin may have differing effects on ischemia as measured by different instruments or provoked by different situations. Specifically, in these preliminary data continuous transdermal nitroglycerin appears quite effective in reducing ischemia detected by ambulatory monitoring during usual daily activities, yet less effective in preventing or delaying ischemia provoked by maximal laboratory exercise.

The ongoing controversy over efficacy of continuous transdermal nitroglycerin for angina may be related to a potential dissociation between nitroglycerin's effect on maximal exercise tolerance (usually measured with laboratory stress testing) as opposed to its effect on the ischemia that occurs with submaximal daily activity (usually measured by ambulatory monitoring). For example, in the largest trial to date of transdermal nitroglycerin for angina pectoris, Muiesan et. al. (9) found a 62% reduction in anginal episodes as determined from patient diaries kept during double blind randomized crossover therapy phases in a subgroup of 29 patients with substantial improvements in exercise time (> 16% improvement over placebo). However, in 23 additional patients with little or no improvement in treadmill exercise time, there was still a 42-48% reduction in anginal episodes during double-blind therapy.

The possibility that transient decreases in coronary flow are involved in the pathogenesis of chronic "stable" angina is not new, having been popularized by Maseri (10) some years ago as "mixed" angina. Several recent studies support the proposition that coronary vasomotion without the dramatic vasospasm that characterizes Prinzmetal's or vasospastic angina may be of considerable importance in many patients with chronic stable angina.

The extensive recent literature on silent ischemia contains considerable evidence that increased myocardial oxygen demands are probably not causal in most cases of silent ischemia. Using ambulatory monitoring, both Schang and Pepine (6) and Deanfield et al (11) have demonstrated that the vast majority of ischemic episodes occur during activities unlikely to increase myocardial oxygen demands, and/or with heart rates much below those causing ischemia on exercise testing. Data from Levy et al (12) using ambulatory pulmonary artery monitoring show that rises in left ventricular end diastolic pressure, presumably a reflection of altered left ventricular contractility and/or relaxation, occur after electrocardiographic evidence of ischemia, and thus are presumably caused by, but are not the cause of ischemia. Similarly, Chierchia et al (13) demonstrated that ischemia as assessed by coronary sinus oxygen tension preceded hemodynamic events (tachycardia, hypertension or increased left ventricular diastolic pressure) as well as electrocardiographic changes, although only five patients were studied and the group was hospitalized with rest angina. Thus, without obvious changes in the determinants of myocardial oxygen demand (heart rate, systemic arterial pressure, or left ventricular contractility) it seems inescapable that many episodes of silent ischemia are likely caused by transient decreases in coronary artery supply.

Variability in the propensity to ischemia at different times of the day is suggested by circadian variations in angina as well as silent ischemic episodes on ambulatory monitoring (14), myocardial infarction (15) and sudden cardiac death (16), all showing peaks in the several hours before 12 noon. That periodic decreases in coronary supply as opposed to increases in myocardial oxygen demands might be responsible for some of these circadian rhythms is suggested by Rocco et al (17), who studied the "ischemic threshold" on ambulatory monitoring, defined as the lowest heart rate during the 24 hour period of monitoring at which electrocardiographic evidence of ischemia was observed. Electrocardiographic ischemia occurred during 26% of instances when heart rate reached the "ischemic threshold" during the morning hours, but only 15% of the time when heart rate reached that same threshold during afternoon hours, implying lower coronary supply in the morning, or more in the afternoon. Direct evidence that coronary artery supply undergoes circadian variation was provided by Fujita et al (18) in twenty-one chronically instrumented dogs with Doppler flow probes implanted on the left circumflex coronary artery and ultrasonic myocardial transducers placed for measurement of length, volume, and contractility indices. In measurements made with awake dogs lying quietly on their sides, there was nearly 13% higher circumflex flow velocity in the afternoon (4 to 5 PM) as compared to the morning, (8 to 9 AM) with no difference in any other hemodynamic parameters.

Various stimuli that commonly precipitate angina are being examined from a new point of view, that of potential reduction in coronary supply rather than increase in myocardial demand. An intriguing study from Winniford et al (19) examined the hemodynamic effects of cigarette smoking in patients undergoing cardiac catheterization. Cigarette smoking caused a 5.6% mean increase in arterial blood pressure while heart rate was held constant by atrial pacing. In patients pretreated with nitroglycerin or calcium blockers, coronary sinus blood flow did increase substantially after smoking a cigarette. In patients not so pretreated, there was no difference in coronary blood flow before and after smoking; given the increased myocardial oxygen demands due to increased arterial pressure, this suggests that smoking caused coronary vasoconstriction which prevented the expected increase in coronary flow. In another study using quantitative coronary angiography, Gaglione et al (20) studied the effects of exercise in angina patients' normal and stenotic coronary artery segments. In normal segments, coronary cross-sectional area increased to 123% of control values with supine bicycle exercise. In stenotic segments, however, cross-sectional area fell to 71% of control values during exercise. Not surprisingly, pretreatment with nitroglycerin prevented this decline in cross-sectional area and indeed caused area to increase even in stenotic segments during exercise. Pretreatment with propranolol unexpectedly had the same effect. The beta blocker, far from causing coronary constriction due to unopposed alpha tone, actually prevented coronary vasoconstriction and produced coronary vasodilation during exercise. What is most interesting about Gaglione's study is the observation that physical exercise, generally presumed to cause ischemia by increasing myocardial oxygen demands, appeared to also decrease coronary artery supply at least in stenotic segments of coronary arteries. Further work is clearly needed as to the mechanism(s) by which stimuli such as cold, emotional upset, or eating produce angina in some patients; it would not be surprising if some or all of these common stimuli for angina exert their deleterious effects by reduction of coronary supply rather than increase in myocardial oxygen demand.

In summary, several lines of evidence now suggest that variations in coronary vasomotor tone play an important role in producing ischemia in several clinical situations. The familiar day-to-day or hour-to-hour variability in chronic "stable" angina might be so explained. For example, it is commonly observed that patients have angina when first arising or with the first exercise of the day (e.g. walking to their car early in the morning), whereas similar or greater exertion later in the day produces no angina. Quantitative coronary angiography has recently demonstrated vasodilation of stenotic segments as well as normal vessels in response to coronary vasodilating drugs, while suggesting that coronary vasoconstriction may be produced by stimuli such as exercise. Circadian variations in the propensity for ischemia, the unequally distributed incidence throughout the 24 hour day of ischemic events such as myocardial infarction and sudden cardiac death, and recent experimental demonstration of circadian variation in coronary blood flow in resting animals all suggest that variations in coronary vasomotor tone throughout the day might not be rare. Finally, although there is as yet no direct evidence, the observed characteristics of silent ischemia are certainly compatible with coronary vasomotion as a cause. Should this hypothesis prove true, the high incidence of silent ischemia among patients with coronary artery disease, and the substantial numbers of episodes of silent ischemia in individual patients with angina both suggest that changes in coronary vasomotor tone are common in the angina population.

Conspicuously lacking in the current hypothesis is any suggestion of what might be causing episodic coronary vasoconstriction or vasodilation. The common occurrence of circadian patterns suggests participation of the central nervous system but whether this is neurologically or hormonally mediated, or occurs by other mechanisms is quite unknown. The high frequency of thrombus in patients with acute myocardial infarction as well as unstable angina invites speculation as to the roles of endothelium, platelets, and the clotting system, but these two clinical syndromes may have quite different pathophysiology from that of chronic stable angina and it is not known whether changing coronary vasomotor tone has anything to do with platelets or the clotting system. What is clear is that substantial efforts need to be directed at documenting, understanding, and eventually preventing disturbances in coronary supply in the large number of patients with what has heretofore been considered demand related angina with "fixed" atherosclerotic lesions. Should derangements in coronary supply prove common, it would suggest reassessment of diagnostic tests for angina. For example, monitoring during activities suggested to frequently produce coronary vasoconstriction (e.g. cold pressor test, mental arithmetic, etc.) might be more appropriate than electrocardiographic recording during bicycle or treadmill exercise, which is specifically designed to increase myocardial oxygen demands. It seems likely that therapeutic options would also undergo reassessment: coronary vasodilators would certainly assume a more prominent role, and increasing attention might well be given to inhibitors of thromboxane, serotonin, platelet active agents, endothelial substances producing vasoconstriction, and the myriad substances, both known and those yet to be discovered, that are likely contributors to coronary vasomotion.

REFERENCES

1. Brunton TL: On the use of nitrite of amyl in angina pectoris. Lancet 2:97, 1867.

2. Murrell W: Nitro-glycerine as a remedy for angina pectoris. Lancet 1:80, 113, 157, 225, 1879.

3. Fye WB: Nitroglycerin: a homeopathic remedy. Circulation 73:21-29, 1986.

4. Brown G, Bolson E, Peterson RB, Pierce CD, Dodge HT: The mechanisms of nitroglycerin action. Stenosis vasodilatation as a major component of drug response. Circulation 64:1089, 1981.

5. Freudenberg H, Lichtlen PR: The normal wall segment in coronary stenosis - a post mortem study. Z. Kardiol 70:863, 1981.

6. Schang SJ, Pepine CJ: Transient asymptomatic S-T segment depression during daily activity. Am J Cardiol 39:396, 1977.

7. Distante A, Maseri A, Severi S, Biagini A, Chierchia S: Management of vasospastic angina at rest with continuous infusion of isosorbide dinitrate. Am J Cardiol 44:533-539. 1979.

8. Shell WE, Kivowitz CF, Rubins SB, See J. Mechanisms and therapy of silent myocardial ischemia: the effect of transdermal nitroglycerin. Am Heart J 112:229, 1986.

9. Muiesan G, Agabiti-Rosei E, Muiesan L, Romanelli G, Pollavini P, Pasotti C, Fiori G, Muratori L, Zuarini AM, Pastorini C, Borziani S, Bozzi LB, Marchetti S. A multicenter trial of transdermal nitroglycerin in exercise-induced angina: individual antianginal response after repeated administration. Am Heart J 112:233-238, 1986.

10. Maseri A, Severi S, DeNes M, et al. "Variant" angina: one aspect of a continuous spectrum of vasospastic myocardial ischemia. Am J Cardiol 42:1019-1035, 1978.

11. Deanfield JE, Shea M, Ribiero P, de Landsheere CM, Wilson RA, Horlock P, Selwyn AP: Transient ST-segment depression as a marker of myocardial ischemia during daily life. Am J Cardiol 54:1195-1200, 1984.

12. Levy RD, Shapiro LM, Wright C, Mockus L, Fox KM: Haemodynamic response to myocardial ischaemia during unrestricted activity, exercise testing, and atrial pacing assessed by ambulatory pulmonary artery pressure monitoring. Brit Heart J 56:12-18, 1986.

13. Chierchia S, Brunelli C, Simonetti I, Lazzari M, Maseri A: Sequence of events in angina at rest: primary reduction in coronary flow. Circulation 61:759-767, 1980.

14. Deanfield JE, Shea MJ, Selwyn AP. Clinical evaluation of transient myocardial ischemia during daily life. Am J Med 79(suppl 3A):18-24, 1985.

15. Muller JE, Stone PH, Turi ZG, Rutherford JD, Czeisler C, Parker C, Poole WK, Passamani E, Roberts R, Robertson T, Sobel BE, Willerson JT, Braunwald E, MILIS Study Group: Circadian variation in the frequency of acute myocardial infarction. N Engl J Med 313:1315, 1985.

16. Muller JE, Ludmer PL, Willick SN, Tofler GH, Aylmer G, Klangos I, Stone PE. Circadian variation in the frequency of sudden cardiac death. Circulation 75:131-138, 1987.

17. Rocco MB, Barry J, Campbell S, Nabel E, Cook EF, Goldman L, Selwyn AP: Circadian variation of transient myocardial ischemia in patients with coronary artery disease. Circulation 75:395-400, 1987.

18. Fujita M, Franklin D: Diurnal changes in coronary blood flow in conscious dogs. Circulation 76:488-491, 1987.

19. Winniford MD, Jansen DE, Reynolds GA, Apprill P, Black WH, Hillis LD. Cigarette smoking-induced coronary vasoconstriction in atherosclerotic coronary artery disease and prevention by calcium antagonists and nitroglycerin. Am J Cardiol 59:203-207, 1987.

20. Gaglione A, Hess OM, Corin WJ, Ritter M, Grimm J, Krayenbuehl HP: Is there coronary vasoconstriction after intracoronary beta-adrenergic blockade in patients with coronary artery disease. J Am Coll Cardiol 10:299-310, 1987.

13

WHAT ARE THE FDA REQUIREMENTS TO OBTAIN A CLAIM FOR THE INDICATION OF SILENT ISCHEMIA?

ROBERT TEMPLE

Director, Office of Drug Research & Review, Food and Drug Administration

Some speakers have not appreciated this, but as Dr. Lipicky said yesterday, we do expect an anti-anginal agent to show an effect on ischemia. Usually, evidence of this effect is derived from exercise testing, but if there are sound ways to do it from Holter monitoring, we would have no problem with that. What is at issue today is whether, and under what circumstances, we would approve a drug solely for an anti-ischemic effect, without evidence of an anti-anginal effect. So far no one has asked us to do this, but there has been an implication today that our failure to have done it already flies in the face of well-established clinical practice, in some way interferes with practitioners' ability to use anti-anginal drugs properly, and is a serious violation of reason and good sense.

The question of whether an anti-ischemic claim could be approved is not purely a regulatory matter; it is similar in many ways to a number of important medical questions that over the years have not been easy to solve. These often turn on whether a documented effect on a surrogate end-point, e.g., an anti-ischemic, cholesterol-lowering, or ventricular premature beat lowering end-point, constitutes an acceptable basis for concluding that the drug has a favorable effect on the "real" end-point, a reduction in mortality or major cardiovascular morbidity. While FDA is often part of these debates because an applicant may seek marketing approval on the basis of the surrogate end-point, it is by no means a situation in which academics all are "pro-surrogate" and FDA is "anti-surrogate". We have come under some criticism at times (although not lately) for not insisting sufficiently on evidence of "real" effectiveness for cholesterol-lowering drugs and we have over the years accepted surrogate end-points for antihypertensive and anti-arrhythmic drugs. Sometimes, I should add, we are "let off-the-hook" by the fact that a drug, while principally used because of a presumed effect on mortality, also provides symptomatic benefits for some people, e.g., as oral hypoglycemics and anti-arrhythmic agents do, and can be approved for the latter claim.

Before considering the anti-ischemia situation I want to consider some of the other instances in which surrogate end-points have been at issue. I also want to point out that physicians can, if they have reason to, use a drug outside the conditions listed in the package insert, and consider some of the examples of this in the past. This is relevant because, at least so far, all of the potential anti-ischemic agents are anti-anginal agents as well and can be made available for that purpose if appropriately studied. Of course, it is possible the anti-ischemic claim would be easier to gain, but the major health question is what a physician's ability to use the drug for silent ischemia would be.

Labeling vs. Practice

It is important to distinguish what occurs in practice from regulatory, labeling, and drug development issues. Practitioners can use drugs as their experience, impressions and conclusions dictate. Anyone wanting to stamp out silent ischemia can do so without waiting for a labeling change. There are many examples of widespread practice that has anticipated changes in labeling, some of them reasonable, some not. Such practices can arise because the literature provides information or speculation that goes beyond labeling; because animal data, or surrogate end-point data, suggest potential benefit, or because of misunderstanding or bad thinking.

Sometimes disparities between practice and labeling are simply a matter of labeling catching up with what is well-established and well-supported by data. The sponsor may be relatively indifferent to adding claims to labeling if he can think of better things to do with research money; the FDA may not put the highest priority on reviewing new claims when there are new chemical entities to look at. Sometimes the pratice is not so reasonable and no application to alter labeling is likely.

Probably the most fundamental reason for disparity between labeling and practice is that evidence of a drug's usefulness for a particular claim does not arise all at once but comes bit-by-bit. The first hints that something is true precede a database that would meet the regulatory standard (or rigorous academic standard - I do not think the two are different) of substantial evidence derived from adequate and well-controlled studies. Some practitioners, through wisdom or luck, may incorporate the new information into practice earlier than others.

In any case, differences between labeling and practice arise fairly often. We do not object to this; indeed, we have no right or reason to object to it. We do not regulate medical practice; we regulate drug companies and claims. Such disparities do, however, deserve attention because they may suggest something we or a sponsor need to look into.

It seemed worth considering a few historical examples of kinds of practice that were or are widespread despite their absence from labeling.

It is well known that propranolol and other beta-blockers were used to treat angina and hypertension long before these claims were approved and added to labeling. If you were to ask the drug companies involved, they would probably say we did not review the data well. If you asked the reviewers involved, they would say the data was not very good and not presented very well. I do not have to resolve that question now, but it is a fact that for almost a decade beta-blockers were used widely outside the package insert. Certainly, in this case, practice was correct in retrospect and the physician using propranolol was doing a wise thing.

Consider another example. I am sure there were people, a decade or more ago, who concluded on the basis of small Scandinavian studies and perhaps the larger, somewhat supportive practolol study, that administering beta-blockers after an acute myocardial decreased mortality. We never received a request to include that claim in labeling, however, until the much more recent timolol and BHAT studies. In retrospect, we know that those early hints were right. Yet at the same time it was quite appropriate that such a claim not appear in labeling because there were insufficient data to support it. Moreover, the consensus of the medical community was that the usefulness of the beta-blockers in that situation needed to be tested fully. That is why some 30 placebo controlled trials comparing beta-blockers and placebo were carried out during this period.

While there was a small group of people who had the right answer before everyone else, it is not a source of embarrassment that the labeling did not reflect what that small group guessed correctly, because the larger consensus was that these were issues that needed to be explored. Even today there is a disparity between labeling and practice. Only three beta-blockers are currently labeled for a post-infarction claim. It is almost certain that the other ones are being used in the same manner, as physicians will extrapolate from one member of a drug class to others and do what they think is right for their patients even if what they do does not appear in the labeling for a drug. I do not find this particularly comfortable, and I dislike the alternatives more. We would either have to assert that post-infarction benefits are a class effect despite no clear evidence of this, or try to dream up studies that would allow the additional agents to gain that claim, which I think is not really possible.

Turning to a third example, recent labeling for antiarrhythmic drugs stresses their role in life-threatening arrhythmias and symptomatic arrhythmias. But I feel certain that there are physicians who continue to use these agents, as they have in the past, to suppress frequent ventricular premature beats (VPBs) in patients without symptoms. In some cases, they have plausible reasons for doing that, even if clear evidence of usefulness is not available. For example, high frequencies of VPBs in a post-infarction setting are plainly associated with increased mortality. And if a physician were to say, "I want to move my patient off one risk curve to the lower risk curve associated with fewer VPBs", they would have a basis for thinking that makes sense. Well, it does "make sense", but there are many reasons to doubt that VPB suppression with available agents, however sensible it seems, is a useful approach. It remains very possible that high rates of VPBs are a marker of increased risk, but not the cause of that increased risk, and that suppressive treatment of VPBs is not of value. To put it another way, VPB rate may not be an adequate surrogate endpoint for judging effects on mortality. Given this, it seems very reasonable for labeling to stress the role of drugs in symptomatic and life-threatening arrhythmias. Physicians may, of course, practice as they choose, but labeling should not accommodate practice unless there is a good scientific basis for it.

Surrogate End Points

The last example is a good introduction to the issue of the acceptability of surrogate end-points. Questions of this kind are rarely easy because, almost by definition, the putative surrogate is plausible, even highly persuasive. Yet there are very good reasons not to be too quick to leap, and the medical community has consistently been prepared to carry out the studies needed to see whether the surrogate was giving the right answer. It seems worth considering some of the situations in which such end-points have, or have not, been evaluated.

1. Heart failure

Heart failure is of interest because it, and especially ejection fraction, is a clear predictor of survival, just as the presence of silent ischemia is. But do we therefore know that moving someone to a new ejection fraction moves him onto a more favorable risk curve? Does it matter what drug you use to improve ejection fraction? We have growing evidence that vasodilators can affect survival in severe congestive heart failure, but it would be a leap indeed to conclude that digitalis, catecholamines, or phosphodiesterase inhibitors would be equally useful, or that any of the agents would be useful prophylactically, i.e., to treat an essentially asymptomatic patient.

2. Anti-platelet drugs

Drugs with demonstrated anti-platelet activity are approved in some countries solely on the basis of evidence of such activity for "diseases in which abnormal platelet function is a problem," whatever people decide those are. We have not been asked to approve that kind of claim, probably in anticipation of what the response would be, and I think it shows how far the surrogate concept can be taken. After all, although there is evidence that aspirin is useful in the post-infarction, unstable angina, and TIA settings, there seems no good way to tell if it is useful in other disease that might be platelet-related (or how to tell which diseases are the result of abnormal platelet function) and no way at all to tell what properties (specific effect, magnitude of effect, and duration of effect) might correspond to, or predict, clinical benefit.

Of course, that does not mean that people who use sulfinpyrazone or dipyridamole, often with aspirin, to prevent stroke, to use after coronary bypass or angioplasty to prevent reocclusion, are wrong. On the other hand, I do not feel that failure or labeling to include such claims is a failing of the system; the state of the data is such that it is not possible yet to say how useful these agents are in those settings.

3. Anti-hypertensive drugs

Most situations in which surrogate end-points are proposed involve prophylactic use of drugs. After all, if a patient is acutely ill, one can fairly readily measure the effect on the illness itself. Surrogates are tempting where the ultimate end-point is hard to measure because it is infrequent and/or far in the future. At the same time, the difficulty is that the gain to the patient is not determined with certainty; you cannot measure a benefit to "lay off" against whatever the adverse effects are. This has been recognized, as I noted above, and the medical community has expanded great effort either to measure the real effect in the first place or at least to find out, after the fact, whether the surrogate was valid.

In the case of anti-hypertensive drugs, many were made available before the concept that drugs need to be shown effective became incorporated into law, and before the idea of controlled mortality studies (or controlled studies of any kind) was established, so there was some catching up to do. It had long been known epidemiologically that hypertension adversely affected survival and this was the principal basis for treatment. In addition, although it is often forgotten, there was, quite early, persuasive evidence of improved survival in patients with malignant hypertension, a condition that had an annual mortality close to 90 percent without treatment. Open studies were persuasive with that kind of historical control.

Despite the epidemiologic and malignant hypertension data there was a strong minority view that hypertension was an appropriate adaptive response to an underlying primary disease and that treatment to lower pressure would lead to devastating end-organ effects: stroke, renal failure and myocardial ischemia. At the time there were no clear data to rebut this, but in the late 60's and early 70's the landmark VA studies showed that treatment of hypertension of moderate to severe degree indeed reduced end-organ damage and major morbidity and mortality.

Therefore, we now, on the basis of the VA studies, epidemiology, and a very substantial consensus, approve new antihypertensive agents on the basis of their effects on blood pressure, secure in the knowledge that for at least some agents, the usefulness of lowering blood pressure is established, and we make no attempt to look at stroke or survival data now. In the absence of such data, however, the drugs are approved for the treatment of high blood pressure without any specific reference in their labeling to what effect that have on survival. If someone were to press the point and want to claim, on the basis of the VA studies, that a new alpha blocker or ACE inhibitor improves survival or reduces stroke, I believe we would resist the idea, as the VA data do not take one quite that far. The only drugs that have really been shown to improve survival or morbidity are reserpine and hydrochlorothiazide and, perhaps, based on more recent data, certain beta-blockers. There is no specific evidence related to ACE inhibitors, calcium antagonists, alpha blockers, methyldopa, etc.

While I believe our current approach is reasonable, the situation is not entirely satisfactory, because there are important unresolved issues. The consistent failure to demonstrate improvement in the outcome of coronary artery disease in hypertension trials is troubling. The MRFIT trial raised a question about whether diuretics, or certain diuretics, could be having an adverse effect on survival. It is reasonable to ask whether drugs that act by very different pharmacologic mechanisms and have different concomitant effects (on heart rate, contractile force, potassium, cholesterol, and triglycerides, for example) all have the same effects on survival and morbidity. Indeed, it is hard to imagine that there is no difference. Yet exploring such questions would require vast resources and, in all probability, what differences there might be would be very difficult to detect. I do not believe it would be reasonable for us to alter our approval standard because of these uncertainties.

Silent Ischemia

Let me now turn specifically to a potential silent ischemia claim. As I noted earlier, the question of whether we accept a silent ischemia claim is not an issue, so far, that affects whether or not particular drugs could be approved or, to any large extent, the speed with which such a drug can be developed. The anti-ischemic drugs, so far, have all been anti-anginal as well and it has not been particularly difficult to gain approval of an angina claim. Some of the data Dr. Scheidt showed before suggest that there may be some capacity to tease anti-ischemic and anti-anginal properties apart. We will have to watch that with interest and adapt to it. As I indicated earlier, labeling a drug for use in angina will not bar the use of the drug for silent ischemia, nor, given the publicly expressed views of some of the people who have spoken today, will a physician doing so have reason to feel he is stepping too far out on a limb and is risking a malpractice action. Finally, as I said before, our current guidelines ask for both evidence of anti-anginal effects and anti-ischemic effects, so that there is no danger that an agent lacking in anti-ischemic effects will somehow slip through as an anti-anginal agent.

What the lack a pure anti-ischemic claim, or a silent ischemia claim does do is prevent pharmaceutical company promotion of this treatment as prophylaxis. I suppose if you believe that silent ischemia is being badly undertreated and that people are suffering because of this, you would consider the absence of such promotion a health loss. But labeling and promotion of drugs is not the only source of advice to physicians, and anyone who believes that silent ischemia is not being sufficiently treated has other means of communicating this.

Let me now turn to what kinds of claims one might consider. A silent ischemia claim could come in two forms: one would be as a supplement to an angina claim, i.e., the drug would be identified as an anti-anginal drug and, in addition, as an agent also good for preventing ischemia even if you do not have angina. Alternatively, one can imagine a primary anti-ischemic claim without any study of actual angina at all.

Let me consider the second of these first. It isn't easy to imagine an agent that affected only silent ischemia and had no impact at all on ischemia accompanied by pain. I think that Dr. Frishman's nifedipine example was interesting but is probably a pharmacokinetic peculiarity and, in fact, it is well known that nifedipine can cause a transient increase in angina as well. Finding that it caused a transient increase in silent ischemia, even if no increased angina was seen in that particular study, is not so surprising.

If a drug were to be worked up only for an anti-ischemia claim, without any attention to the angina situation, what we would have would be an agent potentially useful for angina, indeed, when you really came down to it, probably actually intended to treat angina, but never studied properly for that use. Only ischemia would have been examined, presumably because it is easier to do, or because a drug so studied can be made to seem unique and distinguishable from other drugs. But there are good reasons to consider that an undesirable outcome. First, we really would not know the right dose to be used for treating angina. We do not have a good correlation between an anti-anginal effect and some defined effect on a Holter or on some other measure of ischemia. That does not mean you could not expect that a drug with some effect on ischemia would be effective for angina in some regimen, but you would not know the regimen and you would not know what dose was both effective and well-tolerated.

The nifedipine case to some extent illustrates this. Here you have an agent that is definately effective in angina, as was shown in the study Dr. Frishman cited and in others, and yet has peculiar effects during the day on ST segment abnormalities with, perhaps, an increase early and a decrease late. How would one factor that into a judgment about whether the drug is useful? Does the fact that nifedipine has that effect mean that nifedipine should not be used for angina? It does not, of course, the drug has recognized usefulness in angina. By studying the indirect measure of what you are really after, it seems to me, there is a potential for missing what is more important.

It also seems possible that a drug could have a seemingly favorable electrical effect on some basis other than an anti-ischemic effect. That may not be a worry for the classes of agents we are familiar with, but it seems a potential worry for other kinds of agents, and there does not seem to be a great deal of reason for accepting that risk by failing to study angina.

Finally, it is hard to see what gain can arise from the ostrich-like approach of not studying the claim that really is intended, principally at least, for anti-ischemic agents. In general, where it is reasonably easy to do so, the true intended effect of a drug should be examined, rather than seeking a surrogate that is slightly more convenient but is not in fact the real condition being treated. It therefore seems to me that, as our developing angina guidelines say, anti-anginal drugs should be evaluated for their effect on angina and also for whether they affect ischemia. But ischemia alone does not tell you enough about a potential anti-anginal agent even if, as I will discuss next, an anti-ischemic claim could be itself a valid claim. I offer this conclusion as one suitable for current data where the only clearly established use of an anti-ischemic drug is to treat angina. Information could emerge that would change that and make ischemia a persuasive endpoint in itself.

Let me now consider the question of anti-ischemia as a secondary claim, i.e., as another claim for an anti-anginal agent that has already been properly evaluated for angina. Because no one has actually come forward with a proposed claim of that sort, including well-developed arguments for why it would be reasonable, we have not developed a formal position on it. I feel you get a better idea of what you really think when you hear what a proponent says and I would therefore be most uncomfortable accepting the "con" position, whatever my initial impression, until we had heard the "pro" position fully expressed. I can, however, describe at least the areas of concern that we would have if someone proposed such a claim.

Obviously, as was discussed yesterday, the fundamental question here is whether ischemia is a predictor of mortality because it actually causes or contributes to the risk or because it is a marker for something else that is the real cause of increased risk, such as an abnormality of the anatomy and function of the heart. One should keep in mind a few of the analogous situations I mentioned before, such as increased VPB rates or decreased ejection fraction in the post infarction setting. Both of these are perfectly good predictors of increased mortality. But there is a great deal of uncertainty about whether that is because they cause the problem or reflect some other problem that is the real cause of the risk. Note also that there is considerable logic to the idea that they might actually cause the problem. It is not silly to think that they might be the true cause; it is just that there is a lot of reason to doubt it and no evidence yet for it.

Anyone coming forward with an anti-ischemic claim, it seems to me, would have to be fairly clear about what the putative benefit of this treatment would be. Is it intended to reduce mortality? Obviously, there are no data showing that yet, so that the proposer would have to ask that we, on some basis other than evidence from controlled studies, conclude that is true. What epidemiologic or other information could be brought forth to make the case that treating silent ischemia would enhance survival?

Is treatment of silent ischemia intended to reduce the likelihood of a myocardial infarction? Why should it do that?

Does treatment of non-silent ischemia decrease the likelihood of infarction? Is myocardial infarction the end product of a period of ischemia or is it in fact a different kind of event? I do not want to hide my impression that a persuasive case will be rather difficult to make. It seems important to me that, at least so far, effective anti-anginal drugs, the calcium channel blockers, have not been successful in the post infarction setting in reducing the likelihood of reinfarction or death, a failure that seems not unrelated to the question we are talking about.

Perhaps rather than preventing acute events, prevention of ischemia might, by preventing recurrent ischemic insults, prevent progressive damage and ultimately death due to heart failure, arrhythmias, etc. While one might bring forth arguments to support this, it seems to me one also has to ask whether ischemia might promote development of the collaterals that might be favorable to someone who has an infarction.

Finally, there may be epidemiologic data that could contribute to the case for treating ischemic events. If it turned out that the frequency of ischemia, for patients on or off drugs, was the best determinant of the survival pattern, (i.e., that survival was influenced not by baseline ischemia rate but by the actual rate, whether on therapy or not), that might suggest that you do indeed move someone's risk when you alter his frequency of ischemic episodes; i.e., you move him into a different risk status. Obviously, this kind of evidence needs to be looked at closely, but it is a possible approach.

Anyone proposing prophylactic treatment of ischemic episodes in the absence of a clear effect on survival, would have to deal with the question of weighing long term risk against uncertain benefit. For an extremely safe drug that has a lot of long-term experience, it might be possible to argue that the risk seems so small that it is not something to worry about. In any event, the question would have to be addressed. It seems fairly clear, although even this could perhaps be challenged, that the benefit here is fairly small. Even in the post infarction setting, where continued ischemia is usually present, if you exclude the first few months after an infarction, the use of anti-ischemic/anti-anginal drugs beyond two months has very, very modest effects, if indeed they have any effects at all, on survival. And, as noted, one class of drugs, the calcium channel blockers, so far seems to have no effect at all. So, if you take people who are _not_ in the post infarction setting, and who have a lesser risk, how much benefit can you really expect? Given this, the acceptable risk would seem to be very small.

Finally, I must pose the question, why should one try to _deduce_ the answer to the question of treating silent ischemia, which at best can lead only to endless arguments and no real assurance, when it seems readily possible to carry out trials that can answer the question? If it is accepted, for example, as in Dr. Gottlieb's slide that was shown today, that there is a clear distinction in survival between people who do and do not have silent ischemia, it would not be difficult to design a trial that would show whether a drug that decreased ischemic events by a particular amount had an effect on survival. Surely we are not at a point where we consider it unethical to find out whether long-term treatment of completely asymptomatic people with drugs like calcium channel blockers, which have not been shown to affect survival in any setting, is useful.

What I have tried to do is describe the sort of burdens that someone coming forth with a claim for treating silent ischemia would have to take on. We have not really had an opportunity to consider a full, formal application of that kind, but I think it is clear that the hurdles are not insignificant. It still seems important to emphasize that, as a practical matter, no one is being denied drugs nor the opportunity to practice anti-ischemic therapy if he chooses to do so.

DISCUSSION - 4

Dr. Scheiner: I would like to get down to some real practical issues. One thing in testing angina, we seem to be in a position not to be able to do that very well anymore. There isn't a large supply of anginal patients available to us. There isn't a supply of people that can be placebo controlled anymore and so it seems very odd indeed that we should be trying to evaluate drugs with a symptom limited end point like this that is largely unobtainable today. I think it is probably unrealistic. It also would seem to be the tip of the iceberg. What we have here is we have been testing a group of patients that are at the far end of the spectrum. Their hearts are crying out in pain as an end point when they have had insults that are largely remained undetected up until this point which has been shown pretty well to have produced organic and structural damage to their hearts. I think that has been pretty well demonstrated. Why would anybody want to not prevent these kinds of insults to the heart that are occurring on a repetitive basis. Why would anybody not want to interrupt this spectrum of disease that inevitably ends in a logical fashion with a heart that will fail? Why do we have to wait until we prove that patients that are not treated die this way? I think that is totally unrealistic. It seems to me that what we need from this group today, perhaps the group yesterday are some guidelines as to what would constitute effective treatment for silent myocardial ischemia? Would it be a reduction in the total ischemic time? Would it be reduction in the frequency of it? How would we measure it? Isn't it interesting that even the issue of nitrate tolerance seems to be affected by this. We have suspected for a long period of time that people that are being pushed beyond their level of exertional capacity in order to achieve an unrealistic endpoint and therefore, they can't reproduce it because nitrates for example fall off a little bit in their potency and yet they retain sufficient potency to take care of the major part of the problem of the silent myocardial ischemia. So I think a lot of these points need to be address and why would we as pharmaceutical companies not want to try for labeling changes and all those sorts of things, it is self evident. It is an expensive undertaking to try to get a labeling change for the main purpose of educating doctors out there as to what they should be doing. They need to be informed. They can't be informed when we have restrictions in our labeling, and yet when we don't have guidance as to what we can do in an easy fashion to change that labeling, I think the problem becomes almost impossible to address.

Dr. Morganroth: Let me take the chairman's perogative and break your questions into two different issues. The first is, as Dr. Temple said why would anybody NOT want to focus on angina as an end point in looking at an ischemic claim for a pharmaceutical agent, because that is the principal intent that one will have. What I hear Dr. Scheiner saying is that we can't do that anymore because physicians won't give us angina patients, they will not put them into clinical trials very readily anymore. I would like to hear what the investigators and Dr. Lipicky think. Can we study angina today and is silent ischemia becoming the surrogate end point for these so called angina patients?

Dr. Scheidt: First of all, in terms of how difficult it is to study angina patients, that is absolutely true. The only place in the world where you can get a decent number of angina patients who are willing to have 9 consecutive exercise tests and go on placebo is the Bronx if you are treated by Dr. Frishman. I am sure that every working drug person in this room who has gone to investigators and thousands of bed hospitals finds that you probably have to approach 50 investigators to get 3. They will tell you how many patients they will get, and you should divide that number by 10, and that is the number that you will actually get recruited into the trial. It is a terrible problem and the easy availability of surgery was bad enough, but angioplasty makes the situation impossible, I mean nobody's talking about the malpractice issue, but surely these days, a patient with any significant amount of angina where there isn't something very strange going on, to take that patient off everything for a placebo run ins, and now we are told that our placebo run ins are not long enough that we need a couple of weeks here and there... deep in my heart there may be unusual circumstances where for instance, when calcium blockers were first becoming available, there certainly were some patients who for one reason or another didn't want coronary surgery or couldn't have coronary surgery and they didn't tolerate beta blockers and so they needed a new drug and there you could justify putting them on placebo and running them through all sorts of tests in order to get them on a drug that wasn't available in the United States. That doesn't pertain now. That was the bad news, now let me give you the good news. I don't think it is going to be such a problem at all to prove what one of the things that Dr. Temple said we are ultimately trying to prove. Either we are treating angina or you have to prove that treating silent ischemia really makes a difference and that means survival or prevention of myocardial infarction. I am optimistic about that. You have 3 or 4 trials now in unstable angina where the event rate in the people with silent ischemia is horrendous, horrendous within a very short period of time. People with a good deal of silent ischemia have a substantial event rate over a 20 month period. You don't necessarily have to put people on placebo to show that. All you need to do is observing that there are a group with silent ischemia and after all they are 30-50% people with angina, so there are millions of them out there. There are millions of people with silent ischemia. We need to observe it. We need to get a big group together and I think big group in this case is several hundred patients and I'll bet that within a year or two, you would have substantial differences in event rates. If you don't have that, then I don't know what all the sturm and drung is about because then we are treating a marker and not something real.

Dr. Scheiner: I don't agree with you. I don't think we can do it for silent ischemia any better and I don't think a few hundred patients is going to be sufficient to impress anybody in the process and if it was, that would be a short track to the problem and I wouldn't be standing up here now.

Dr. Morganroth: Let's ask Dr. Lipicky and then Dr. Temple if an application came in with not just a simple change in the marker but a clear demonstration in one trial that was well correlated and conducted that demonstrated a decrease in death and/or myocardial infarction if that would be sufficient for a claim.

Dr. Scheidt: Not placebo controlled. Everybody on therapy but a group with silent ischemia versus a group without and perhaps different types of treatments. I was backing it up into a more asymptomatic but take an unstable angina in the trial design you just described, would that be sufficient to approve a drug.

Dr. Lipicky: I want to respond to your first question also. I guess at the last cardiorenal advisory committee meeting, there was a single mortality trial in class 4 congestive heart failure that involved less than 200 patients and it resulted in a claim for survival. Certainly an appropriately designed trial that would have a terrifically statistically significant result and had been properly conducted, etc. etc. certainly would be paid attention to. It seemed to me that if you took people with three vessel disease who had silent ischemia at least looking at some of the curves that were shown yesterday it is not clear to me that it would take a lot more patients than that. Can I return to your first question because there are two things that are probably appropriate to say. We recently had been involved in a large anti-anginal trial with transdermal products and I guess over the course of two years there have been some 500 people who have been enrolled in that trial not that that was easy or that it didn't take a number of large centers over a reasonable period of time. These people were being asked to enroll in a trial where I think that over the course of the trial, there were something like 36 exercise tolerance tests that were being performed, so it can be done, one. Secondly, we have just recently completed, but the data is not analyzed yet, a study of all of the applications that had been submitted to FDA that involved randomized placebo controlled background medication free, exercise tolerance anginal trials in order to look at the drop outs due to any kind of cardiovascular event and/or death. The data is not completely analyzed, so I can't tell you what it says, but I have seen the raw numbers and I can without any problem say that there certainly isn't the slightest suggestion in the data that placebo was a problem. The end point being cardiovascular events including mortality and there just isn't a hint that placebo is bad. Sometime in the next six months or so, I think we will have completed the analysis and we have looked at everything ever submitted to the FDA.

Dr. Scheidt: One thing that immediately comes to mind is that the groups that are in these trials are a very unusual type of angina patient and indeed they are the people, all of whom have reproducible stress tests within narrow guidelines, 10 or 15%. They are undoubtedly the people who have the most demand related angina. They are the minority of patients on that screen with those German investigators who have knocked the coronary artery with the eccentric lesion which is the majority of patients. They are the very small group who have concentric lesions, who have not a lot of vasoconstriction and vasodilation and I mean that is fine, except that is not the universe of angina patients. It is like everybody criticizes the CASS study because the CASS study screened 15,000 people in the registry and ended up randomizing 700 and those are NOT really representative of the universe. It is the same thing here. The people who get in these very small drug studies, that finally get done, and that take 4 years and 59 centers to do. Every investigator knows that he saw 1000 people with angina during the time it took to recruit 5. Of the 995, more representative or are the 5? The people in these drug studies are unusual patients. Some of them are relatives of Dr. Frishman. Some of them are people I have known a long time who are unbelievably stable and that is why placebo is O.K. in those patients. It is a different group of patients and I am really worried. Sure we do what is required by the drug companies, by the FDA and everybody is very careful about it and obviously you need objective data, but there is this voice deep down saying I am selecting such a small group of unusual people for the drug trials, are they really representative of the universe?

Dr. Temple: It seems to me Bill Frishman gave part of the answer to that before which is that when you look, at least in most settings, the non-painful episodes seem to drop off roughly in parallel and the drugs that have been tested and approved by these mechanisms seem to be both anti-ischemic and anti-anginal. I am not sure that people who give stable responses to exercise testing are necessarily people who are stable all day. It may just be that they do have some particular fixed lesion that gets them when they exercise. It is not clear how unrepresentative they are. I should also add that in days gone by when there were more people who were allowed to have angina without having an operation, the same studies used to measure anginal attack rates and exercise tolerance in any individual, the response on angina attack rate did not necessarily correlate terribly well with exercise tolerance, but drugs that affected one always affected the other. You had the feeling that given the diversity of human behavior from day to day, you didn't always get a 1:1 correlation but that they were in fact measuring much the same thing. Painful episodes of course. They were not at that time measuring painless episodes. The system seems to work O.K. The ideal that it is hard to study this doesn't necessarily suggest that it is the right solution because you still want to be sure that you have a drug that works in angina. You may want to be sure about other things as well, but you do want to know that. I don't understand how someone could say based on present data, just what electrocardiographic Holter finding corresponds to an effective anti-anginal agent. I sympathize with the difficulty of trying to find the patients. It probably had something to do with the fact that there are available therapies and people are reasonably satisfied with them, but that doesn't suggest what the solution is. If you want to work up a drug for angina, it doesn't seem possible to avoid studying angina. I should add that the reason exercise tolerance is now so prominent compared to anginal attack rate, is that people with significant attack rates are hard to find except in the Bronx and so we have tended to rely on people who have a very small number of events per week where it would be very difficult to show reduction of events and rely on exercise tolerance because even though they have few events they do have some load that stimulates angina.

Dr. Scheidt: We are not disagreeing at all. I couldn't agree more. Drugs shouldn't be approved on the basis of changes in ST segments, but my solution to that is that you need to show changes in morbid events. I am relatively optimistic because you have plenty of people with silent ischemia out there and I think it should be a good marker, is it really going to be that difficult to show changes in morbidity-mortality?

Dr. Cohn: Of course if we could predict with 100% accuracy what the results of multicenter trials which have yet to get started in many places would show would be quite helpful. I tend to agree with you. I would think that in the triple vessel disease group that we are going to be able to show down the road a bit some of these changes that people have indicated. I think the questioner and others are asking, why do we have to stand on our heads in a sense to do this. I have to get back again. We have talked about the fact that looking at a stable angina population with very low event rate etc, we don't know that they have very few ischemic episodes. We know they have few episodes of angina. Just simply for example in doing away with the exercise test, using the Holter monitor, when everyone is happy with the technology and showing that Joe has one episode of angina a week and 10 episodes of silent ischemia and your drug is not only relieving the angina but also done away with a lot of the other ischemia would allow the drug company to make the claim that they have an anti-ischemic preparation and an anti-anginal preparation and never have to get near the exercise test for example. There is one drug company that I have seen advertisements for in fact, one of the makers of verapamil that have been advertising the fact that their drug based on studies like this is effective for angina and is effective for silent ischemia. It says it in their advertisements. You said you react to these things. What has been your reaction to that? It has been running for 6 months.

Dr. Temple: I don't necessarily read the same journals you do.

Dr. Cohn: That is a non-answer.

Dr. Temple: I think that has to be looked at closely. You have to read what the words say and what the level of claim is and people can offer little bits of information without making an overt claim. I can't say because I haven't seen it.

Dr. Scheidt: But Peter don't you agree that there ought to be something beyond numbers of changes of ST segments. That you ought to try at least for the the morbidity-mortality and it shouldn't be too hard to find.

Dr. Cohn: I agree, but when we reduce anginal episodes, no one asks us to produce morbidity and mortality figures for that. That is the point I am making. I think there is a consistency. The FDA has got in this angina mold and to reset it in terms of modern technology and approach is very difficult and I keep on making the point that 5 years from now. I made this point yesterday when we talked about hypertension and MI's. When it is obvious that treating ischemia is good. It helps the heart. The heart should not be ischemic. We will look back and say gee it was obvious back in 1987, I wonder what took those guys so long to realize it.

Dr. Temple: I am not sure why it is so self evident. It seems perfectly legitimate to ask what you are seeing is a marker of something that is going to lead to trouble or because of the trouble itself. What is wrong with my examples of VPB rates greater than 10. What more logical connection could there be than something that you see like that and sudden death?

Dr. Cohn: A VPB is simply an electrical instability. We don't know, and we can't make the connection between that and sudden death unless you have a statistical..

Dr. Temple: That is because we are smarter now and we know that. Everybody thought you could before.

Dr. Cohn: We could show that a portion of the heart is not receiving no adequate perfusion, its wall motion is inadequate, it is producing lactate, it is functioning in an abnormal way, that is different from saying that there is an electrical signal of which we are not really sure what it means. The heart is being damaged during ischemic events. Fortunately most of the time its transient, just like with angina. You have seen enough evidence. We have all seen enough evidence that some of these episodes are prolonged. We have to make the next jump and show you that prolonged LV dysfunction, prolonged metabolic alterations will eventually lead to bad things happening to the heart and when we do that, we will say, gee that is fine and this makes sense and interventions probably can help that. What we are saying is on the face of it, and the question we are asked is why is it so illogical to not allow the heart to be rendered ischemic? What is the logic of that?

Dr. Lipicky: In part the illogic of that is that you are ascribing the ischemic events and their repeated occurrence to something bad that happens to the patient and that is the logic that is behind that. It could be that the repeated ischemic events are simply a manifestation of the advancing coronary artery disease and that it is really the coronary artery disease that is going to culminate in the event of an MI or death and that that is not in fact related to the number of times there are ischemic events and you are associating the natural history of the coronary artery disease process saying that if you can detect that the transient and ischemic events are changed in their frequency that that is a reflection of changing the natural history of the disease and you don't know what the relationships are.

Dr. Cohn: We do remember from yesterday all the nice data showing those subgroups. That the determinants of mortality were going to be the extent of vessel disease, the extent of LV function and the amount of ischemia. I think Don Weiner showed that very nicely. Others have shown the same thing for the same amount of vessel disease and LV dysfunction and the patients with more ischemic events on exercise tests, on Holter, call it what you will are going to have the worse outcome. Therefore the logic would go the other way. The logic would say if we reduce the ischemic events, perhaps we are going to impact favorably. Now it is not proven. We are just talking about the logic here. The logic would argue that rather than the other way around that the ischemia has nothing to do with it.

Dr. Temple: What about improving ventricular function? Would the logic say that doing that would be good too?

Dr. Cohn: Yes, logic would say that if you could reduce the cause of the LV dysfunction, you would be able to help the patient. If the LV is totally scarred, we know we have a problem, but if the LV is dysfunctional because of muscular abnormalities that are coming as a result of ischemia and by reversing this, we might be able to show improvement. There were studies done several years ago and were still done and in fact in terms of mortality, that showed that if you could demonstrate there was viable myocardium left in a heart with coronary disease, and we did some of them with post-extrasytolic potentiation and catecholamines etc, that that persons mortality was lessened over the long run with medical or surgical therapy. The theory being that if there is viable muscle there, there is something that can be salvaged so it would mean translated today, that any attempt we can make to salvage viable muscle, and you know we do that with heart attacks, should be attempted. That is the logic. I think that is what the question was trying to say, if I phrased it incorrectly. That is the logical approach is to try to do this.

Dr. Temple: What evidence would you advance to say that those episodes themselves cause permanent damage to muscle?

Dr. Cohn: The only evidence that we have is of course indirect. We have autopsy studies in people who have never had a documented myocardial infarction by history or by ECG, who have never had a clinical history of angina for that matter. These are Bill Roberts studies who come to autopsy because of sudden death and at autopsy, the heart shows evidence of scars, evidence of previous small infarctions as well as extensive atherosclerosis. So the supposition is that these people, even though they haven't any symptomology, have had repeated bouts of damage to the heart which directly or indirectly has lead to their demise. To make the 1:1 assumption of course Bob, I can't make that except for those anecdotal stories of people wearing Holter's. They get ischemic without symptoms and they go ahead and die, but those are anecdotal stories. I agree with Steve that as we collect more data especially in our symptomatic populations who also have silent ischemia, these truths will become in a sense self-evident in the years to come, but the argument keeps on coming back to the beginning. What is the harm in a drug being advertised as being anti-ischemic as well as anti-anginal? We'll forget the just anti-ischemic for the moment, but why can't both be used?

Dr. Frishman: I don't think we have any complaint with that. Again, the point I made is that the drugs that we have that have been shown anti-ischemic and anti-angina most of them wouldn't you agree Peter would be anti-ischemic even when there is no pain. Silent ischemia is the real entity and I think it needs to be treated, but just like angina, we know we can reduce angina or ischemic episodes, but we at least haven't proven that we can prolong life yet, and therefore it may turn out that in the study where we look at the silent ischemia in the treatment versus non-treatment, we may actually find out we don't do anything on survival. Although it is an entity it may all go to worse prognosis. The therapy may in fact do nothing. It may turn out that all we can really do with anti-ischemic drugs is reduce pain and we can't do anything really to change the natural outcome in patients. That is why I think that the study that Steve did is so important and I think that will address a lot of questions. I would be the first one to say that if one could show, and I think that people with silent ischemia are going to do worse, but if one could show that a drug is going to change the natural history. That is an important thing.

Dr. Cohn: The point I am making Bill is that these kinds of studies are going to be ongoing and we are going to have an answer for this in 4 or 5 years when the studies are organized etc. My point is why argue form the pessimistic point of view and say that maybe 5 years down the road they'll show now effect which they might. They also might show an effect. Why must we wait 5 years using that argument, that's all. We have objective ways of showing that ischemia is going to be bad. We are treating patients for ischemia. There is no question we do. We have drugs available, we treat them. I have a question about this because I have been using calcium blockers and beta blockers to treat totally asymptomatic individuals and we are going to be publishing our results soon and they are going to show very dramatic decreases in ischemia.

Dr. Scheiner: This is another issue entirely, but we can't go into a doctor's office and give him any information outside of our own labeling. We are in a kind of catch 22 situation because we can't get the change in the labeling unless we know how to get the change in the labeling and unless it is a realistic possibility without doing some kind of huge studies with mortality end points. The net effect of all of this, the information doesn't get out there beyond you gentlemen to where it should be going and benefitting the public and I think that is the bottom line.

Dr. Scheidt: Let me come to the FDA's defense. First of all it is not a trivial issue because I do not think that we know that you should treat silent ischemia and if we advertise it to the whole world, the drug bill goes up by billions of dollars and we will all get more flack from the administration, they will freeze medicare fees etc. etc. This is not a trivial issue. If you don't need to treat silent ischemia, you ought not be advertising and suggesting that it be treated. I must admit that although I think deep in my bones that silent ischemia will turn out to need treatment, I don't think anybody can say today, should be treated. There are 20 million episodes of silent ischemia a week in the United States. That is my guess, there are 4 million patients with angina and everybody with angina maybe has 3 episodes of angina a week on average, so they have 4 times as many episodes of silent ischemia, not everybody, half of them have silent ischemia so that is 2 million who have silent ischemia out of the 4 million and each one has 3 painful so that means about 10 or 15 non-painful... it is millions of episodes a week in the United States. In most cases, and after all this silent ischemia all around us, the mortality-morbidity rates from coronary disease are falling substantially. Now maybe it is because patients are being treated for angina and therefore they are also being treated for silent ischemia. I really do think that before we go off and treat many more people much more vigorously, you need to show that you are doing something to it and I think that it ought to be possible very quickly. I do not think that it has to take 5 years because you are going to have much higher rates of change and at least the preliminary data is that it is a good marker. If you have a good marker that shows you a high risk group, just as in the congestive failure where the mortality rates are high, you can show something relatively quickly with reasonable numbers of patients.

Dr. Morganroth: Dr. Lipicky was that a sufficient defense or do you want to comment further?

Dr. Lipicky: Just two other thoughts and I am not sure I will say them right, but it seems to me that the argument of having a claim approved in order to be able to educate practicing physicians is not a very compelling argument. I don't think it should be our responsibility to prove claims so that physicians can be educated. That doesn't seem like it is a very powerful argument. The second aspect of that same kind of thought is that, at least as I understand scientific method, there is somebody's picture of how the universe functions, which ordinarily would be called hypothesis, that the scientific method says that the hypothesis is worthy if it can be formulated in some way that allows it to be tested and verified. Then if it turns out that the hypothesis doesn't have the predictive value expected, then one modifies the hypothesis appropriately. The hypothesis that is being forwarded sounds to be perfectly sound, and perfectly rational and perfectly valid. Because it is a sound, valid hypothesis, does not mean it is true, at least not as I understand the scientific method and it needs to be verified and if it is not true, it needs to be modified and it seems to me that that is how things work. It sounds to me that it is much ado about nothing.

Dr. Temple: It seems hard for me to imagine that all drugs will behave the same way, if there is a benefit to be attained, it is hard for me to imagine that all drugs will behave in the same way. I presume anyone who values reducing silent ischemia is now shaken to the roots and is going to avoid nifedipine because the total ischemic burden isn't reduced in that setting. But I don't think that would be a logical thing to do, but if you follow the rules, those little excesses at the beginning presumably are very dangerous. Do we believe that? Probably not. There are many things to find out. Some drugs may have larger effects on those than others. Some may have transient effects because they have short half lives and there will be escape. Usually what you have is some hypothesis as Ray says and then there is some kind of epidemiologic data that makes people believe in the hypothesis and then folks argue about that is good enough or should there be a controlled trial. At this stage, we really don't even have the epidemiology, the strong suggestion that you can move people along to a different curve. Maybe someone could assemble data of that kind now, I don't know, but we didn't really see that yesterday. What we have is a description of a phenomenon. A marker of high risk, I want to come back to it. It is highly logical to think or it would have been 10 years ago to think that if you found VPB rates associated with high mortality suppressing them ought to work. That is the most logical thing in the world. We know better now because it doesn't seem to have worked out because people have studied it and found that the hypothesis didn't...

Dr. Morganroth: That has not been studied properly, we don't know that.

Dr. Temple: O.K. You don't like the studies yet and maybe that is so but it turns out in those settings where you are not sure of the benefit that side effects become important, even trivial ones, so a small increase in lipids that a drug might cause might be enough to overcome the benefit. You can't know those things until you do something with the bottom line.

Dr. Cohn: Let me just make one point earlier, you mentioned about the nifedipine study. The work from England originally showed that when nifedipine was given in 30 mg doses there was a significant drop in the total ischemic episode and angina and that when combined with propranolol it was even better and in our studies in which we have used 30 mg dosages in asymptomatic patients indicate the exact same thing, a dramatic 50% reduction in event rates. I think that Bill Frishman's study and I am sure he would agree himself and he has said so using tremendously high doses of nifedipine as monotherapy is really not a valid way of looking at that medication. Secondly, while we are on the subject of calcium blockers I noticed that you never referred and the fact that anti-ischemic medications, you said only have been shown in the post-infarction, the beta blocker, what about the diltiazem and the non-Q wave study? Isn't that another indication of an anti-ischemic drug having a beneficial effect?

Dr. Anders: There seems to be a lot of emphasis from the FDA and Dr. Temple that in order to get a least a secondary approval for silent ischemia one will have to show some kind of outcome with respect to survival or morbid events and I am asking why do we have to do this or is there emphasis on that when for years we have been selecting and probably introducing a selection bias selecting angina patients to reduce angina frequency, nitroglycerine consumption, etc. etc. to show efficacy. Can we go ahead like Dr. Peter Cohn and not stand on our head but just show efficacy and then maybe go ahead and look at survival. If we are going to show efficacy, what would the investigators and the FDA be comfortable with as a minimum or adequate set of monitoring techniques, i.e. treadmill tests, Holter monitoring, or radionuclide assessment?

Dr. Morganroth: We will hold the second part of that because that is the same second question that Dr. Scheiner raised that I have held off. The principal issue is do you need to show impact on mortality over morbidity for an approvable claim versus just the end point. I think that has been debated.

Dr. Lipicky: The question is why is that different from angina and I think no one has addressed that. It seems to me that one wants to make an approval based on knowing that there is some kind of clinical benefit in an area where the state of the art is not such that one is simply willing to buy a pharmacological effect as sufficient and if one can affect a patient's symptomatology. The reason that the patient comes to the doctor is that the patient wants some help and that is sufficient justification it seems to me to say that if one can show that one has affected that phenomenon that that is fine. Whether one knows that there is a long term outcome or not, the patient has a complaint and with this medicine the doctor can help the patient. If the patient has no complaint and the doctor is going to make the patient have two headaches a day in order to have some projected benefit that no one has measured, how do you do that risk benefit assessment? So it is different and there needs to be some benefit shown, because the benefit is not included in the documentation that the drug works, whereas if one can show an effect on anginal pain, the benefit is included in the basic observations.

Dr. Morganroth: Unless the benefit is relief of documented ischemia which immediately has a deleterious effect on the ventricle.

Dr. Anders: Not only that, but control of angina itself has not shown to improve survival or control morbid events.

Dr. Cohn: We know now why. Probably we are not controlling all the ischemic events.

Dr. Lipicky: It is the analgous circumstance to what one would not hesitate to prescribe an analgesic for someone who had a headache because they had a brain tumor that was expanding even though one know that one had absolutely NO hope of influencing the brain tumor. The patient needs some care and that is a perfectly reasonable thing to do. If the reason for giving the medication for the headache is to make the brain tumor go away, it that is the reason for giving the medication, one would certainly want to see evidence that the brain tumor is going away and I think that if one says if I prevent repeated ischemic events, that that is good for you, there has to be some documentation that it is. If one says that I am giving the medication to relieve the pain or to allow you to walk farther before you get the pain so your level of activity can increase to some degree, that you have objectively demonstrated that the patient is being benefited with that very same measurement. That is the difference.

Dr. Temple: The proof positive that something changes mortality is not the only conceivable way of learning something. There are other kinds of evidence that can be deduced. I mentioned that in connection with lipid lowering agents. The case here doesn't seem overwhelmingly persuasive. More important it seems to me that people are not paying attention to the fact that these drugs are not entirely benign. They all have occasional side effects. We don't have a lot of long term data on most of them, but they have the usual panopoly of side effects people have. It is odd to me for example, that people spend a lot of time thinking about the consequences of being on a beta blocker in the post-infarction setting and they talk about how many people you have to treat to save just one, how dismal it is to be on one. The side effects in that setting are quite well recognized. We know verapamil causes constipation, nifedipine does that, they are not completely benign drugs. It is not necessarily a pleasure to be on one. It affects your life. There ought to be some reason to decide to put someone on life-long therapy and in the absence of a pretty persuasive case, it doesn't seem suitable to do it. I come back to the anti-arrhythmic thing. A lot of people got put on quinidine for valid logical reasons and it probably didn't do a lot of them much good and probably worse. It seems to me there is the possibility of reproducing that kind of error unless people pay attention as early as possible to the nature of what the real benefit is, which I must say seems a very reasonable thing to do before drugs are labeled rather than after.

Dr. DiPalma: We are looking at the whole subject of ischemia as being a defect in plumbing or maybe a defect in action potentials and we are not looking at it as a biochemical lesion and certainly the knowledge of what happens to the myocyte when there is ischemia is very extensive. The point is that it is interesting that in Europe they are treating the ischemia as a biochemical lesion. For example, aconitine combats or eliminates the collection of free oxygen radicals which are very destructive to the myocyte. People are taking this. In fact I think there is a popular book written about it which the public reads and uses. It is amazing to me that none of this has been mentioned and is an approach. The question is, would it be a valid claim as far as the F.D.A. is concerned to investigate a drug which corrects a biochemical defect of ischemia.

Dr. Frishman: We have in fact looked at co-enzyme Q-10 in the Bronx and it has been looked at in New Orleans and Oklahoma and in fact it turned out to be anti-anginal, so that the observation that this may have unique anti-ischemic properties, it turns out that the drug may actually turn out to be an anti-anginal drug also, although those studies may need to be confirmed.

Dr. Morganroth: What is the mechanism of its action?

Dr. Frishman: It is an interesting drug, we have no idea.

Dr. Morganroth: Does it effect vasomotor tone?

Dr. Frishman: We don't know. This was just a clinical study. It is used in Japan for the treatment of heart failure, so again, that shows how much you really know about ischemia and angina. There may still be even other classes of agents yet unknown that in fact may be working but this needs to be corraborated. It turns out it is not just a pure anti-ischemic drug that in fact has an equivalent anti-anginal effect.

Dr. Lipicky: Do you remember we have seen that. Somebody here who works with us ought to know what it does. It gets into the cell somehow and is indeed a co-enzyme and is one of the major circles.

Dr. Frishman: It is ubiquitous. It works in the mitochondria and it is involved in ATP. The question is the mechanism by which it works in angina, but it is involved in oxyphosphorlization It is an important co-enzyme step there and allegedly in certain patients there is a deficiency of this and if you place it it might really make a difference, but this is really being looked at. In health food stores, a dose of coenzyme Q is subtherapeutic so if people run out now and use it, it really is not the dose you have to use in practice.

Dr. Morganroth: That is another subject for another day as to how some of these things that look like pills and are taken as pills in fact as drugs tend to be distributed as food stuffs and therefore they are not regulated in the same way.
Dr. Temple: The difficulty with a biochemical change is that it isn't always easy to know what the biochemical change means. I guess if people can develop a strong case that you are talking about a fundamental mechanism, you can start thinking about those things, but there are so many materials that have been alleged to affect metabolism in one way or another that it seems to me a very difficult thicket to sort your way through. What seems appropriate to me is to ask what benefit is this supposed to accomplish and then study it.
Dr. Morganroth: Let's move on to recommendations about study methodology. I was impressed by the data that when you look at the frequency of silent ischemic episodes, that they are not reduced by 90% or better, but only by about 50% on treatment. Being experienced in the PVC area with new 1C antiarrhythmics, we would expect a potent drug to get rid of most of these markers like a 99% median reductions. I always thought that the beta blockers and calcium channel blockers were reasonably good anti-ischemic medications particularly in combination and I wonder why we are not seeing a better reduction in the number of silent ischemic episodes? What kinds of criteria should be used in terms of duration or number of episodes and what percent reductions should be required? Is Holter recording sufficient?
Dr. Cohn: In exercise induced silent ischemia, the same guidelines should apply that apply for painful exercise induced ischemia. You want to prolong the time at which you get your ischemia. It is very unusual to negate it completely as we all well know, but you can delay its time of onset. You can minimize the amount of ST segment depression that you see or the thallium defects, etc. But eventually you will got them, but you can delay this and you can let people enjoy an ischemia free day just as you would an angina free day. However, when it comes time to reducing the amount of episodes per day or the duration, we know a couple of things. We know based on the variability studies that Selwyn and Deanfield have done independently that you have to reduce the episodes at least in a large group of patients at least 50% to make a claim, and I don't want to use claim in the FDA sense, to make a statement that your drug is effective. I think for monotherapy, the nitrates, the beta blockers and the calcium blockers already have and will be shown to be able to do that as monotherapy. But to try to get the level down to 0, I think you are going to have wind up with a combination of drugs. I think the goal is to reduce total ischemic activity to as much near nil as you can, just as you can with episodes of VT for example as best as you can. Then this is our goal in terms of clinicians who treat ischemia, forget silent ischemia, just ischemia. Whether we can translate this into improved morbidity and mortality, that is our goal and we are going to try and prove it and that is the way we are going to try and do it, by having treatment arms that will reduce ischemia as close to 0 as possible. Our control groups will be people who have been

treated, because you can't put anybody on placebo anymore as you know, who have not had a reduction to that degree.

Dr. Temple: I guess I am not sure I understand why you can't have in fact have a placebo group of a kind. You could randomize patients to two different policies, one of reducing their anginal event rate or of extending their exercise tolerance. Another group could be randomized to a tremendous push to try to eliminate as many ischemic events as possible.

Dr. Morganroth: Same drugs in both arms?

Dr. Cohn: I can't put a patient ethically on placebos for long periods of times. One arm can be usual care, and the other arm could be intensive care.

Dr. Temple: Or if you are correct in your guess there, your conclusion is that monotherapy is not going to really reduce the total ischemic load all that much and that you are going to use combinations, so that one group could get monotherapy and the other group could have something else.

Dr. Cohn: Of course, but I think we have to show that each type of drug, the nitrates, the beta blockers, the calcium blockers and all the different permutations are effective as monotherapy. That is why I thought his particular study was very misleading because of the dosage and that reflex tachycardia.

Dr. Temple: You could in fact imagine three major trials and I don't know how big they would have to be. That would depend on the mortality and event rate in the population, one of which used a member of each of the three classes, the other of which added to that class the other agents and you could then learn whether any benefit is agent specific, you would have the opportunity to factor in pharmacokinetic effects.

Dr. Cohn: Everything depends on the event rate in the groups obviously and where we do have a problem. When you have an end point of only MI's or death, those are very hard end points and once a patient breaks through his medication and develops unstable angina, or worse than angina goes to angioplasty and surgery, they are a loss to your study. We are going to lose patients unless we can make unstable angina requiring hospitalization as another end point for example.

Dr. Lipicky: It should. That is an end point.

Dr. Temple: What can get studies of this kind going. I don't hear that that kind of thing is happening yet.

Dr. Cohn: There is only one thing that we need. We have the organizational basis already.

Dr. Temple: Let me guess.

Dr. Cohn: It starts with M and ends with Y.

Dr. Frishman: I would agree with Peter that you look at silent ischemia and we'll be looking at it the same way we look at anginal episodes. Single drugs to see if they reduce episodes, double drugs to see if they work better than single drugs in that capacity and the model that we have used for angina efficacy was single and combination therapy on hold in evaluating these transient ischemic changes. The other possibility for why we don't eliminate all these ischemic episodes and most of the studies that have been done where one tends to become pain free on therapy and still has residual ischemia maybe not all the episodes are related to coronary dysfunction. In fact maybe the background that occurred may be a lot of variability. In fact we are dealing with some episodes of false positives.

We may in fact not be accomplishing the goal by reducing it by 50%.

Dr. Cohn: If we can show one group is reduced 90% and the other group is only reduced 30%, but morbidity and mortality are favorably affected, that would make the case.

V. COMBINATION DRUG THERAPY—FDA ISSUES

14

COMBINATION DRUG THERAPY: WHAT STUDIES ARE REQUIRED TO OBTAIN APPROVAL?

RAYMOND J. LIPICKY, M.D.

Director of the Division of Cardio-Renal Drug PRODUCTS OF THE FDA

In my view, the development of combination products should proceed concomitantly with the development of new chemical entities since, for the same investment, one can get two products marketed with the same effort. Current practice is to develop just the new chemical entity and, after it is marketed, doing a whole other set of trials that develop a combination product. There is a lot of room for improvement in combination product development.

The general operant policy for approval purposes is that a combination product must show that each of the active ingredients contribute to the effect of the combination. The database that is submitted in support of a combination product NDA needs to contain data that show that. As you will see, there are other things that probably one should keep track of also.

For discussion, consider the development of an agonist/antagonist combination. One ingredient produces an undesirable effect, an agonist, and the other one counteracts that undesirable effect, an antagonist. The classical example would be hydrochlorothiazide and triamterene. What one would want to know in a circumstance of that sort is that for a given dose of Drug A (agonist) that produces a given intensity of side effect, (e.g. hypokalemia) what should the dose of Drug B (antagonist) that would maximally counteract the side effect. A trial design that would enable one to address that issue would be to start a population on Drug A until one had the side effect and then to randomize the population that had the side effect to placebo and varying doses of Drug B. In that way one would be able to say for a dose of A, I need this much B. If one wanted to have more than one dose of A, for each dose of Drug A one would have to randomize varying doses of Drug B again. After deciding upon the doses of A and B one would need to take the combination product, as developed, and do another study that showed that nothing funny happened when that combination was actually used in practice. Depending on the circumstance, one might want to do some other things, but all of this appears straightforward conceptually.

The real issue comes where one has two drugs that produce the same effect and, for the sake of discussion lets deal just with anti-hypertensives. Think of an ACE inhibitor and thiazide as being the models that we will discuss.

The most historically prominent approach is to take a population of hypertensive persons and start them out on Drug A (or even take them while they are already receiving Drug A) and randomize from that population those patients who are considered to be unresponsive to Drug A. In that randomized population add Drug B or a placebo. This would indicate that Drug B has an effect when added to A; therefore, one could conclude that Drug B contributes to the effect of Drug A. It would be nice to have something up front here to show that Drug A actually had an effect, but as far as approvability is concerned, that has not been a requirement.

One must also define the converse by taking another population, start it out on Drug B, take the people who are unresponsive and randomize them to Drug A or placebo. These two trials, together, would satisfy the statutory requirement of two or more controlled trials and would be taken as evidence that A plus B is better than A or B.

There are still a number of problems with such a development plan, though this has been a basis of approval for a large number of drug combinations. For example, one is that if one chooses a beta-blocker and a thiazide and enrolls a population of all black people for the beta-blocker-add thiazide study, and a population of all white people for the thiazide-add beta-blocker study, the results of the two trials would be consistent with the conclusion that A&B is better than A or B. Yet, no individual who received the combination would in fact have had an effect from both components.

Therefore, from such designs one's ability to extrapolate is limited. There is no dosing information that can be derived.

All one can possibly conclude is that at the top of the dose response curve, those Drug A and Drug B are probably additive. To execute such trials one would need at least 160 patients enrolled for each study. We have seen new drug applications for combination products that employed designs of this sort with as many as 1,500 patients enrolled in controlled clinical trials and did not develop sufficient information to support approval.

Another way of approaching the problem is to bring people into trial on placebo then randomize the population to placebo, Drug A, Drug B or a combination of A & B (a 4 armed parallel trial). At least that solves one problem, all people are randomized at the same point so there is no selection bias. One has an estimate of the effect of A, an estimate of the effect of B and one can say whether A plus B is better than A or B. So, that is a little better from the vantage point of generalizability. But, indeed, it still provides no dosage information. It is only applicable in one setting. There is still only one conclusion you can draw and that is that the 2 drugs are additive and individuals in the population may not have an effect from both drugs.

A third way of approaching the issue of combination therapy is to do what has been called a multifactorial design trial. Data from such a trial has been presented before by Eli Lilly in public so I do not think I am giving away any secrets. This was a study of pinacidil and hydrochlorothiazide. What was studied was 12.5 mg, 25 mg, and 37.5 mg of pinacidil and 12.5 and 25 mg of hydrochlorothiazide. Each dose of each agent was studied alone and in combination. Placebo was present as a control. A total of only 384 patients were studied, about the same number as in the start on A add B, start on B add A trial designs.

There were interpretable results that are of interest. The first result that is of interest is that pinacidil did show a rate limiting side effect (edema) and one can plot the pinacidil doses that were used on one axis and the hydrochlorothiazide doses used on another axis and the incidence of edema on a third axis. One can easily see that the incidence of edema was a function of not only the dose of pinacidil but also the dose of hydrochlorothiazide. Not surprising, but such data would simply not be available as a result of either of the previously discussed designs.

Looking at such three dimensional response surfaces, one can derive more insight regarding how the two drugs interact in addition to concluding that A+B is better than A or B. For example, the evolution of the time course of blood pressure response can be seen. The entire response surface evolves over the whole eight weeks of the trial so that the information during the first period of the constant dose level is not quite the same as the information that one gets at the end of the trial.

One of the major problems with a successful implementation of this design is the range of doses that one includes (the number of doses that clearly cost in sample size and the range of the doses that are studied). In this particular trial, I would have liked to see a wider range of doses studied of both compounds. Provided that a response surface was developed, I would be perfectly willing to interpolate, not extrapolate but interpolate, between actual data points to make decisions about what kinds of dose or what the dose of each ingredient should be. One cannot write such instructions for use from any of the previous designs.

The last thought, we have not thought that titrated trials are very useful from the vantage point of dose ranging. They rather consistently (and I think that has been proven by subsequent studies) lead one to the wrong estimation of dose if handled by conventional statistical data and interpreted in conventional ways. But, if one applies some non-linear mixed effects modeling to data from a titrated trial (assuming that an effect must go from zero to some maximum effect and making the assumption that the effect is a continuous and monotonic function of dose) then indeed one can take data from titrated ascending dose trials and, in reasonably small populations, determine reasonable estimates of ED50s that do not disagree remarkably from the estimates that come from parallel dose ranging trials.

One could do that for one using each subject as their own control and because of the analysis tool that is being used (preserving the identity of individuals within the estimate of what the drug did in that individual). Using different analytical tools, one can get away with studying only a couple of dose levels in each individual, a couple of combinations of levels in each individual, and can probably accomplish dose ranging of four or five doses of each of two drugs and of each dose in combination from studies that are no bigger than 300 or 400 total.

Of course there is little experience with the latter two designs, but combination drug development does have some interesting things associated with it that I related to experimental design and data analysis. Approaches discussed can contribute information with respect to not only the development of a combination product but would be expected to, if done at the same time a new chemical entity is being developed, support approval of the new drug with a more appropriate choice of the unit dose of the new chemical entity and also support approval of a combination product.

SYMPOSIUM ON NEW DRUGS AND DEVICES

OCTOBER 15 & 16, 1987

PARTICIPANT LIST

Erik Agner, M.D.
Med. Dept. B / University State Hospital
Blegdamsvej 3, DK-2100
Copenhagen O
1 39 66 33

Pablo I. Altieri, M.D.
Professor of Medicine
Director of Cardiovascular Labs
University of Puerto Rico
School of Medicine
GPO - Box 5067
San Juan, Puerto Rico 00936

Robert J. Anders, Pharm.D.
Regional Medical Manager
E.R. Squibb & Sons
P.O. Box 4000
Princeton, NJ 08540
(201) 359-9709

Melody Anderson, M.S.
Senior Clinical Research Associate
Syntex/Institute of Clinical Medicine
3401 Hillview Avenue
Palo Alto, CA 94303
(415) 496-3508

Vidya S. Banka, M.D.
Chief, Division of Cardiology
Episcopal Hospital
Front Street & Lehigh Avenue
Philadelphia, PA 19125
(215) 427-7247

John M. Barden
Senior Clinical Research Associate
Stuart Pharmaceuticals
Concord Pike & New Murphy Roads, OW2
Wilmington, DE 19897
(302) 575-2634

Joachim Baumann, M.D.
Bayer AG, 5600 Wuppertal - 1, Fed. Rep. Germany
Pharma Research Center, Clinical Research II
Aprather Weg
0202/368524

C.L. Beach, Pharm.D.
Scientist, Clinical Research
Marion Laboratories, Inc.
P.O. Box 9627
Kansas City, MO 64134
(816) 966-5000

Mirza Beg, M.D.
Vice President, Medical Affairs
Smith, Kline & French
1500 Spring Garden Street
Philadelphia, PA 19101
(215) 751-6376

Joseph R. Bianchine, M.D., Ph.D.
Vice President, Medical Research and Development
DuPont Critical Care
1600 Waukegan Road
Waukegan, IL 60085
(312) 473-3000

Selvyn Bleifer, M.D.
Director of Cardiology
HCA Brotman Hospital
414 N. Camden Drive
Beverly Hills, CA 90210
(213) 278-3400

Sharon L. Bonney, M.D.
Associate Director, Medical Research
Miles Pharmaceuticals
151 Deerfield Drive
Hamden, CT 06518
(203) 937-2281

Agnes A. Bouvet, M.D.
Director
CIBA-GEIGY
556 Morris Avenue
DEV 3054
Summit, NJ 07901
(201) 277-5784

Dennis J. Bowsher, M.D.
Associate Clinical Pharmacologist
Lilly Lab for Clinical Research
Wishard Memorial Hospital
1001 W. 10th Street
Indianapolis, IN 46202
(317) 276-4797

Dr. Charles Boyle
F. Hoffmann-LaRoche & Co. Ltd.
Dept. PKF/TK, B.1407/52
CH-4002
Basle (Switzerland)
(061) 27 59 69

Ellen M. Brady, M.D.
Associate Medical Director
CIBA- GEIGY Pharmaceuticals
556 Morris Avenue
Summit, NJ 07901
(201) 277-7255

Betty Brisse, M.D.
Med.Klinik der Univ.,
Albert-Schweitzer-Str. 33
44 Munster
West Germany
0251/837621

Linda M. Brown
Senior Research Specialist
Cardio Data Systems
56 Haddon Avenue
Haddonfield, NJ 08033
(609) 354-2222

Robert S. Brown
Senior Research Specialist
Cardio Data Systems
56 Haddon Avenue
Haddonfield, NJ 08033
(609) 354-2222

Walter Brownsberger
Marion Laboratories, Inc.
9300 Ward Parkway - West 2
Kansas City, MO 64114
(800) 821-2130

Brian S. Bryzinski, M.D.
Associate Director of Clinical Research
Lederle Laboratories
Middletown Road
Pearl River, NY 10965
(914) 732-3030

Larry Bush, M.D.
Research Fellow
Merck Sharp & Dohme Research Laboratories
West Point, PA 19486
(215) 661-7828

C. Cabot, M.D.
Director
Cardiovascular Clinical Research
CIBA-GEIGY Corporation
556 Morris Avenue
Summit, NJ 07901
(201) 277-5373

Rita A. Carey, Ph.D.
Smith Kline & French Laboratories
1500 Spring Garden Street
Philadelphia, PA 19101
(215) 270-6306

Dr. Peter Chan
Group Leader
Cardiovascular Biological Research
Medical Research Division
American Cyanamid
Pearl River, NY 10965
(914) 735-5000

Sughok K. Chun, M.D.
Medical Reviewer
Food and Drug Administration
HFN-110, Room 16B45
5600 Fishers Lane
Rockville, MD 20857
(301) 443-0320

William A. Clementi, Pharm.D.
Associate Director
Lorex Pharmaceuticals
4930 Oakton Street
Skokie, IL 60077
(312) 982-8413

Marc D. Cohen, M.D.
Vice President/Cardiovascular Drug Development
CIBA-GEIGY
Pharmaceuticals Division
556 Morris Avenue
Summit, NJ 07901
(201) 277-5874

Roy Collins
Product Manager
ICI Pharma
16 Falconer Drive, Mississauga
Ontario L5N 3M1 CANADA
(416) 821-8000

Judith Cubbon
Associate Medical Director, Cardiovascular
Apt. 7A, 10 W. 66th Street
New York, NY 10023
(212) 873-7276

Barbara Curtis, R.Ph.
The Upjohn Company
301 Henrietta Street
Kalamazoo, MI 49001
(616) 385-7841

Ellen E. Dempsey
Clinical Research Scientist
Nordic Laboratories
16700 TransCanada Highway
Kirkland, Quebec H9H 4M7
(514) 694-9690

Robert G. Dempsey, III
Manager, Corporate Pharmaceutical
New Product Planning
Eli Lilly and Company
Lilly Corporate Center, Bldg. 74/5, MC501
Indianapolis, IN 46285
(317) 276-4433

Anthony DePadova, M.D.
Director, Medical Affairs
CIBA-GEIGY Corporation
556 Morris Avenue
Summit, NJ 07901
(201) 277-5408

Philip L. Dern
Medical Officer
Food and Drug Administration
HFN-110
5600 Fishers Lane
Rockville, MD 20857
(301) 443-0319

Norma Dias, M.D.
Senior Associate Medical Director
Dept. of Clinical & Scientific Affairs
Pfizer Pharmaceuticals
235 E. 42nd Street
New York, NY 10017
(212) 573-3105

Robert DiBianco, M.D.
Associate Clinical Professor of Medicine
Georgetown University School of Medicine
7600 Carroll Avenue
Takoma Park, MD 20912
(301) 891-5485

Joseph R. DiPalma, M.D.
Emeritus Prof. Pharmacology & Medicine
Hahnemann University School of Medicine
Broad and Vine Streets
Philadelphia, PA 19102
(215) 448-3470

Robert K. Dix, Ph.D.
Associate Director
Pfizer
235 E. 42nd Street
New York, NY 10017
(212) 573-7329

Douglas N. Dobak
Manager, Regulatory Affairs
DuPont Pharmaceuticals
Barley Mill Plaza
Wilmington, DE 19899
(302) 992-3593

Gisela Doring, M.D.
c/o E. Merck, Clinical Research Division
P. O. Box 4119, 6100 Darmstadt
06151/72-3293

Dr. Peter Dumovic
Product Director
CIBA-GEIGY Pharmaceuticals Div.
556 Morris Avenue
Summit, NJ 07901
(201) 277-5864

David A. Dworaczyk
Project Manager
E. I. DuPont de Nemours & Company, Inc.
Barley Mill Plaza, P25-2177
Wilmington, DE 19898
(302) 992-2408

S. Edwards
Senior Clinical Research Scientist
CIBA-GEIGY Corporation
556 Morris Avenue
Summit, NJ 07901
(201) 277-5008

Stewart J. Ehrreich, Ph.D.
Senior Technical Advisor
Biometric Research Institute, Inc.
1401 Wilson Blvd.
Arlington, VA 22209-2306
(703) 276-0400

Charles A. Ellis, M.D.
140 Haverhill Street
Andover, Mass. 01810
(617) 470-0966

Maria Erdelyi-Brown
Managing Editor - Clinical Symposia
CIBA - GEIGY
14 Henderson Drive
West Caldwell, NJ 07006
(201) 882-4795

Dr. Dale B. Evans
Associate Director Pharmacology
Sterling-Winthrop Research Institute
81 Columbia Turnpike
Rensselaer, NY 12144
(518) 445-8109

J. L. Fischetti, M.D.
Senior Associate Director
ICI Americas
Stuart Pharmaceuticals
Wilmington, DE 19897
(302) 575-2038

T. J. Fitzsimmons, M.B., Ch.B., MRCP
Therapeutic Area Team Leader
Medical Research Department
ICI Pharmaceuticals
Mereside, Alderley Park, Macclesfield
Cheshire SK10 4TG, England
(0625) 582828 Ext. 3760

Michele R. Flicker, M.D.
Director of Medical Affairs
Marion Laboratories, Inc.
P.O. Box 9627
Kansas City, MO 64134
(816) 966-5000

Jeffrey J. Freitag, M.D.
Director, Clinical Research
Wallace Laboratories
Half Acre Road
Cranbury, NJ 08512
(609) 655-6806

Jeffrey Friedman, M.D.
Wyeth Laboratories
P.O. Box 8299
Philadelphia, PA 19101-8299
(215) 688-4400

M. Fujimori, M.D.
Director, Clinical Investigation (Japan)
American Cyanamid Company
Medical Research Division
Lederle Laboratories
Pearl River, NY 10965
(914) 735-5000 Ext. 2406

Gary A. Gemian
Senior Product Manager
Key Pharmaceutical
2000 Galloping Hill Road
Kenilworth, NJ 07033
(201) 558-4576

Fredric R. Gerber, M.D.
Senior Associate Medical Director/Group Leader
Pfizer Laboratories
235 E. 42nd Street
New York, NY 10021
(212) 573-3590

Thomas P. Gibson, M.D.
Director, Clinical Research Cardiovascular
Merck Sharp & Dohme Research Laboratory
10 Sentry Parkway
Blue Bell, PA 19422
(215) 834-2645

Pritam Gill-Kumar, M.D.
Food and Drug Administration
HFN-110
5600 Fishers Lane
Rockville, MD 20857
(301) 443-0319

Kenneth M. Given, M.D.
Executive Director, Regulatory Affairs
Merck, Sharp & Dohme Research Laboratories
West Point, PA 19486
(215) 834-2315

John C. Godfrey
Associate Director of Clinical Research
Rorer Pharmaceuticals
800 Business Center Drive
Horsham, PA 19044
(215) 956-5031

Hector J. Gomez, M.D., Ph.D.
Senior Director
Merck Sharp & Dohme Research Laboratories
WBD-236
P. O. Box 2000
Rahway, NJ 07065-0914
(201) 750-8031

Leonard M. Gonasun, Ph.D.
Director, Medical Research
Sandoz Pharmaceuticals
Route 10
East Hanover, NJ 07936
(201) 386-7850

Dr. Paul G. Gooding
Director, Clinical Research
Product Acquisitions
American Cyanamid
Game Cock Island
Greenwich, CT 06830
(914) 732-5000

Maryann Gordon, M.D.
Assistant Director, Cardiovascular-Renal
Hoechst Roussel Pharmaceuticals, Inc.
Route 202-206 North
Somerville, NJ 08876
(201) 231-2998

Juan R. Guerrero, M.D.
Vice President, Medical Research
Knoll Pharmaceuticals
30 N. Jefferson Road
Whippany, NJ 07981
(201) 428-4150

Jeffrey Granett
Associate Director, Clin. Investigation
Smith, Kline & French L-221
P.O. Box 7929
Philadelphia, PA 19010
(215) 270-5660

Dr. Gary Grover
Research Investigator
Squibb Institute for Med. Research
Pharmacology Department, F4135
P.O. Box 4000
Princeton, NJ 08543-4000
(609) 921-4733

B. J. Harlow, M.D.
Senior Medical Advisor
Syntex Clinical Research Europe, Spur House
23-25 Marlow Road
Maidenhead, Berkshire, SL6 1RD, U.K.
Maidenhead (0628) 72211

Linda Harver, RPH
Regulatory Affairs Specialist
Eastman Pharmaceuticals
9 Great Valley Parkway
Malvern, PA 19355
(215) 640-8731

Anthony Helstosky
Clinical Research Associate
Sterling-Winthrop Research Institute
81 Columbia Turnpike
Rennselaer, NY 12144
(518) 445-8994

Sharon A. Henry, M.D.
Medical Director
Princeton Pharmaceutical Products
P.O. Box 4000
Princeton, NJ 08543-4000
(201) 359-9721

Elaine J. Hinsch
Clinical Project Coordinator
Hoffmann-LaRoche Inc.
340 Kingsland Street
Nutley, NJ 07110
(201) 235-3351

John N. Hurley, M.D., Ph.D.
Assistant Vice President & Medical Director
Medical Department
Ayerst Laboratories
685 Third Avenue
New York, NY 10017
(212) 878-6953

Mr. Hiroshi Ishikawa
Project Manager
1251 Avenue of Americas
New York, NY 10020
(212) 582-0008

Yasmin Islami
Manager, Cardiovascular Portfolio Management
Ciba-Geigy Pharmaceuticals Division
556 Morris Avenue
Summit, NJ 07901
(201) 277-5329

Robert E. Keenan, M.D.
Medical Officer
Food and Drug Administration
Cardio-Renal Division
HFN-110, Room 16B45
5600 Fishers Lane
Rockville, MD 20857
(301) 443-0319

Donald Jeffrey Keyser
Manager, Product Approval
Marion Laboratories, Inc.
P. O. Box 9627
Kansas City, MO 64134
(816) 966-5062

Harold J. Kissell
President
Medical Education Programs, Ltd.
372 Danbury Road
Wilton, CT 06897
(203) 834-1811

Knud Knudsen, M.D.
Medical Officer
Food and Drug Administration
Cardio-Renal Division
HFN-110, Room 16B45
5600 Fishers Lane
Rockville, MD 20857
(301) 443-0319

Norman W. Lavy, M.D.
Vice President & Senior Adviser on
Medical & Regulatory Affairs
E.R. Squibb & Sons, Inc.
P.O. Box 191
New Brunswick, NJ 08903
(201) 519-2941

Robert J. Lee, Ph.D.
Vice President, Research & Development
DuPont Critical Care
1600 Waukegan Road
Waukegan, IL 60085
(312) 473-3000

Jan N. Lessem, M.D., Ph.D., FACC
Clinical Research Section Head
Syntex
3401 Hillview Avenue
P.O. Box 10850
Palo Alto, CA 94303
(415) 852-1945

Ronald Lieberman, M.D.
Staff Medical Officer
Food and Drug Administration
Cardio-Renal Division
HFN-110, Room 16B45
5600 Fishers Lane
Rockville, MD 20857
(301) 443-0319

Earle Lockhart, M.D.
Medical Director
Glenbrook Labs
12 E. 86th Street
New York, NY 10028
(212) 907-2764

Ib Bo Lumholtz, M.D.
Medical Director
Sandoz Ltd., Titangade 9A
DK-2200 Copenhagen N
1 83 61 02

Lisa Ann Luther
Clinical Research Associate
Hoffmann-La Roche Inc.
340 Kingsland Street
Nutley, NJ 07110
(201) 235-3419

Dr. Garry Macdonald
Head of Cardiovascular
Clinical Research Group
BAYER UK LTD
Bayer House, Strawberry Hill
Newbury Berkshire RG13 1JA
England
(0635) 39313

Daniel J. MacNeil, M.D.
Associate Medical Director
Miles Pharmaceuticals
400 Morgan Lane
West Haven, CT 06516
(203) 937-2339

Hans Mader
Assistant Director
Cardiovascular Business Development
Sandoz Pharmaceuticals
Route 10
East Hanover, NJ 07936
(201) 386-7843

George E. Maha, M.D.
Executive Director, Clinical Research
Merck Sharp & Dohme Research Laboratories
West Point, PA 19486
(215) 834-2635

Sara Armstrong Mahler, M.D.
Group Director, Cardiovascular Diseases
DuPont Pharmaceuticals
Barley Mill Plaza - P26/1278
Wilmington, DE 19898
(302) 992-4674

Richard D. Mamelok, M.D.
Associate Medical Director
Syntex
P. O. Box 10850 - A3-288
Palo Alto, CA 94303
(415) 354-7205

Harold K. Marder, M.D.
Director, Clinical Research
Wyeth Laboratories, Inc.
P.O. Box 8299
Philadelphia, PA 19101-8299
(215) 341-5792

Peter R. Maroko, M.D.
Group Director
Cardiovascular/Renal Products
Smith Kline and French Laboratories
E43
1900 Market Street
Philadelphia, PA 19101
(215) 751-6378

Dr. Irwin G. Martin
Director, Regulatory Affairs
Smith Kline & French Laboratories, F20
1500 Spring Garden Street
Philadelphia, PA 19101
(215) 751-3835

Mark N. Matthews
Product Manager
CIBA-GEIGY
Summit, NJ
(201) 277-5320

Frank McBarron, M.D.
Director, Cardiovascular Research Dept.
Chiles Research Institute
Providence Medical Center
4805 NE Glisan
Portland, OR 97213
(503) 230-6011

Raymond McCoy
DOREMUS PORTER NOVELLI
888 Seventh Avenue
New York, NY 10106
(212) 315-8121

Robin McGarry-Myers, M.D.
Assistant Director, Clinical and Medical Affairs
Stuart Pharmaceuticals
Concord Pike & New Murphy Roads
OW2
Wilmington, DE 19897
(302) 575-8209

Alan B. Miller, M.D.
Chief of Cardiology
University Hospital of Jacksonville
Division of Cardiology
655 W. 8th Street
Jacksonville, FL 32209
(904) 350-6598

Edgar W. Mitchell
Manager, Product Registration/Approval
Marion Laboratories, Inc.
Marion Park Drive
Kansas City, MO 64137
(816) 966-5000

Dr. Donna Moisey
Assistant Director
Pfizer
235 E. 42nd Street, REA Bldg.
New York, NY 10017
(212) 573-1531

Dr. Lisa Monsen
Associate Medical Director
Pfizer
235 E. 42nd Street, REA Bldg.
New York, NY 10017
(212) 573-1218

Maria J. Montenaro
Clinical Research Associate
Sterling-Winthrop Research Institute
81 Columbia Turnpike
Rensselaer, NY 12144
(518) 445-8858

Kevin M. Mullane, Ph. D.
Director, Cardiovascular Research
CIBA-GEIGY Pharmaceuticals
Summit, NJ 07901
(201) 277-4673

Michael Muro
Senior Research Specialist
Cardio Data Systems
56 Haddon Avenue
Haddonfield, NJ 08033
(609) 354-2222

Diana Nichols
Asst. Business Development Manager
Smith Kline & French Laboratories
1500 Spring Garden Street
P. O. Box 7929
Philadelphia, PA 19101
Mail Code E-77
(215) 751-7513

Dr. R.-E. Nitz
Cassella AG
Hanauer Landstr. 526
D-6000 Frankfurt/Main 61
GERMANY

Patricia L. Neubert
Product Manager
CIBA-GEIGY Corporation
556 Morris Avenue
Bldg. D-3058
Summit, NJ 07901
(201) 277-7128

Carolyn O'Connor
Vice President of Drug Research
Services Division
Clinical Data, Inc.
1172 Commonwealth Avenue
Boston, MA 02134
(617) 734-3700

Janet V. Okopski
Medical Information Manager
Lorex Pharmaceuticals
Old Bank House, 39 High Street
High Wycombe, Bucks HP11 2AG
England
0494/26188

Robert I. Outwater
Director, Cardiovascular Regulatory Affairs
Ciba-Geigy
556 Morris Avenue
Summit, NJ 07901
(201) 277-5599

Alfred F. Parisi, M.D.
Chief, Cardiology
VA Medical Center
1400 VFW Parkway
West Roxbury, MA 02132
(617) 323-7700

Vincent S. Parziale, M.D.
Clinical Investigator
Eli Lilly and Company
Lilly Corporate Center
Bldg. 31/4, MC622
Indianapolis, IN 46285
(317) 276-3659

Jillian R. Pincus, M.D.
Associate Medical Director
Sandoz Pharmaceuticals
59 Route 10
Building 501-1
East Hanover, NJ 07936
(201) 503-8814

John R. Plachetka, Pharm.D.
Associate Director, Clin. Invest.
Glaxo Inc.
5 Moore Drive
Research Triangle Park, NC 27709
(919) 248-2445

David Poorvin, Ph.D.
Director, Cardiovascular Research
Schering Corporation
2000 Galloping Hill Road
Kenilworth, NJ 07033
(201) 298-4538

Dr. W. John Powell, Jr.
Executive Director, Clinical Research
Merck Sharp & Dohme
BL 3-3
West Point, PA 19486
(215) 834-2583

Cheryl J. Priest, R.N.
Medical Research Associate
Eastman Pharmaceuticals
9 Great Valley Parkway
Malvern, PA 19355
(215) 640-8728

Robert F. Reder, M.D.
Director, Medical Affairs
Knoll Pharmaceuticals
30 N. Jefferson Road
Whippany, NJ 07981
(201) 428-4170

Robert Reynolds, Ph.D.
Associate Clinical Research Director, Cardiovascular
Beecham Laboratories
501-551 5th Street
Bristol, TN 37620
652-3101

Lair Ribeiro, M.D.
Executive Director
Ciba-Geigy
Summit, NJ 07801
(201) 277-7414

Richard L. Riley, Ph.D.
Associate Director of Clinical Research
Rorer Central Research
800 Business Center Drive
Horsham, PA 19044
(215) 956-5030

Ms. Susan Rinne
Group Manager
Syntex Corporation
M.S. A2-250
Palo Alto, CA 94034
(415) 855-6117

Marilyn J. Rogers
Regulatory Affairs Manager
DuPont Pharmaceuticals
Barley Mill Plaza
Med. Products Dept. P27-2322
Wilmington, DE 19898
(302) 992-5451

Martin Rose, M.D.
Group Leader for Antihypertensive Drugs
Division of Cardio-Renal Drug Products
HFN-110
Food and Drug Administration
5600 Fishers Lane
Rockville, MD 20857
(301) 443-0319

Hans J. Rosenbach
Director, Transdermals, Medical Affairs
CIBA - GEIGY
Summit, NJ 07901
(201) 277-5656

Alberto Rosenberg, M.D.
Vice President, Clinical Research
Wallace Laboratories
P. O. Box 1
Cranbury, NJ 08512
(609) 655-6325

Lois B. Rosenberger, Ph.D.
Research Leader
Hoffmann-LaRoche Inc.
340 Kingsland Street
Nutley, NJ 07110
(201) 235-3957

A. A. Rubin
Director, Sci Info & Technol
DuPont Pharmaceuticals
Barley Mill Plaza
Wilmington, DE 19898
(302) 992-4657

Ewa J. Rucinska, M.D., Ph.D.
Director
Merck Sharp & Dohme
Research Laboratories BL 3-1
West Point, PA 19486
(215) 834-2642

Dr. Robert R. Ruffolo, Jr.
Group Director
Department of Pharmacology and
Department of Molecular Pharmacology
Smith Kline & French Laboratories
P.O. Box 1539
King of Prussia, PA 19406-0939
(215) 270-6050

Janet E. Rush, M.D.
Director, Clinical Research-Cardiovascular
Merck Sharp & Dohme Research Laboratories
West Point, PA 19486
(215) 834-2648

Magdi Sami, M.D.
Associate Professor of Medicine
Royal Victoria Hospital
687 Pine West
Rm. M476
Montreal - Quebec H3AIAI
(514) 842-1231 ext. 350

Stuart L. Scheiner, M.D.
Director, Cardiovascular
Wyeth Laboratories
King of Prussia Road
Radnor, PA
(215) 341-2987

Dr. Wolfgang Schulz
Medical Director
Cassella AG
Hanauer Landstr. 526
D-6000 Frankfurt/Main 61
(069) 41 09-2265

Richard P. Schwarz, Jr., Ph.D.
Director, Cardiovascular Program
Sterling-Winthrop Research Institute
Renssalaer, NY 12144
(518) 445-8390

Ms. Ilona Jupina Scott
Regulatory Associate
Smith Kline & French Laboratories, F20
1500 Spring Garden Street
Philadelphia, PA 19101
(215) 751-3836

Dr. David G. Shand
Senior Vice President
Janssen Research Foundation
40 Kingsbridge Road
Piscataway, NJ 08854
(201) 524-9456

William Shapiro, M.D.
Professor of Medicine
University of Texas Health Sciences Center
Cardiovascular Section
4500 So. Lancaster Road
Dallas, TX 75216
(214) 372-7906

Wayne C. Shaw
Medical Program Coordinator
Merck Sharp & Dohme Research Laboratory
10 Sentry Parkway
Blue Bell, PA 19422
(215) 834-2652

David Sheps
Associate Professor
338 Clinical Sciences Bldg.
229-H
Chapel Hill, NC 27514
(919) 966-4215

Steven A. Silber, M.D.
Associate Director
Cardiovascular/Renal Products
Smith Kline & French Laboratories
E43
1900 Market Street
Philadelphia, PA 19101
(215) 751-6378

Dr. L. Silver
Assistant Director
Pfizer
235 E. 42nd Street, REA Building
New York, NY 10017
(212) 573-1418

Mark A. Sirgo, Pharm.D.
Associate Director
Glaxo Inc.
5 Moore Drive
Research Triangle Park, NC 27709
(919) 248-2193

Lynne Smith
Account Representative
Clinical Data Inc.
1172 Commonwealth Avenue
Boston, MA 02134
(617) 734-3700

Jonathan B. Solsky, M.D.
Research Physician
Hoffmann-La Roche Inc.
340 Kingsland Street
Nutley, NJ 07110
(201) 235-2043

John Somberg, M.D.
Associate Professor of Medicine and Pharmacology
Albert Einstein College of Medicine
Bronx, NY 10461
(212) 436-3566

Ole Helmer Sorensen, M.D.
Med. Dept./Sundby Hospital
DK-2300 Copenhagen S.
1 55 15 55

Joseph Souhrada, M.D.
Associate Director, Cardiovascular Dis.
Pfizer
Eastern Point Road
Groton, CT 06340
(203) 441-5026

Lester F. Soyka, M.D.
Therapeutic Area Clinical Director
Cardiovascular Research
Bristol Myers Company, PRDD
P. O. Box 5100
Wallingford, CT 06492-7660
(203) 284-6838

Joan Standaert
Food and Drug Administration
30847 E. River Road
Terrysburg, OH 43551
(419) 259-6211

Peter H. Stone, M.D.
Assistant Professor of Medicine
Harvard Medical School
164 Longwood Avenue
Boston, MA 02115
(617) 732-1604

Steve G. Svokos, Ph.D.
Vice President, Regulatory & Technical Affairs
Knoll Pharmaceuticals
30 N. Jefferson Road
Whippany, NJ 07981
(201) 428-4012

Charles S. Sweet
Senior Scientist
Merck Sharp & Dohme Research Laboratories
Department of Pharmacology - W26-208
West Point, PA 19486
(215) 661-6517

Colin R. Taylor, M.D.
Pfizer Inc.
Director, Clinical Research Department
Eastern Point Road
Groton, CT 06340
(203) 441-4807

Jim Teasdale
Cardiovascular Specialist
Key Pharmaceuticals
620 Williams Avenue
Runnemede, NJ 08078
(609) 931-8891

Martin J. Thoolen, Ph.D.
Research Pharmacologist
E. I. duPont deNemours & Company
Medical Products Department, E400/5412
Wilmington, DE 19898
(302) 695-7300

Pieter B. Timmermans, Ph.D.
Manager, Cardiovascular Science
E.I. du Pont de Nemours & Company, Inc.
Medical Products Department, E400/4257
Wilmington, DE 19898
(302) 695-7188

Samuel A. Tisdale, Jr., M.D.
Director, Clinical Research
A.H. Robins Company
1211 Sherwood Avenue
Richmond, VA 23220
(804) 257-2801

Heino Trees, M.D.
Medical Officer
Food and Drug Administration
Cardio-Renal Division
HFN-110, Room 16B45
Rockville, MD 20857
(301) 443-0319

Julio Tubau, M.D.
Director, Hypertension Research
VA Medical Center
4150 Clement Street
San Francisco, CA 94121
(415) 221-4810

John Tuckman, M.D.
Associate Medical Director
Medical Department
Ayerst Laboratories
685 Third Avenue
New York, NY 10017
(212) 878-5981

Lorin A. Wagner, Ph.D.
Associate Medical Director
Schering Corporation
2000 Galloping Hill Road
Kenilworth, NJ 07033
(201) 298-4664

Janice Wahl, M.D.
Senior Associate Director of Clinical Research
Boehringer-Ingelheim Pharmaceuticals, Inc.
P. O. Box 368
Ridgefield, CT 06877
(203) 798-4201

Penelope Walsh
Medical Research Associate
Miles Pharmaceuticals
400 Morgan Lane
West Haven, CT 06516
(203) 937-2290

David P. Ward, M.D.
Director, Cardiovascular Products,
International Medical Affairs
Smith Kline & French, C17
1500 Spring Garden Street
Philadelphia, PA 19101
(215) 751-3413

Edmund L. Webb, M.D.
Rorer Central Research
Building 1
800 Business Center Drive
Horsham, PA 19044
(215) 956-5032

Dr. Roger Wheywell
Medical Director
BAYER UK LIMITED
Bayer House, Strawberry Hill
Newbury Berkshire RG13 1JA
(0635) 39313

Th. Widmann, M.D.
Hoffmann-LaRoche PkF/Tk
Grenzachersti 124;CH-4002
Basel, Switzerland
61-278031

John W. Williams, M.D.
Associate Medical Director
Sandoz
27 Zeck Road
Morris Plains, NJ 07950
(201) 503-7685

Park W. Willis, III, M.D.
Chief, Section of Cardiology
B-208 Clinical Center
Michigan State University
East Lansing, MI 48824
(517) 353-4830

Phillip M. Young, Pharm. D.
Senior Clinical Research Scientist
Marion Laboratories, Inc.
P. O. Box 9627
Kansas City, MO 64137
(816) 966-5000

GPSR Compliance

The European Union's (EU) General Product Safety Regulation (GPSR) is a set of rules that requires consumer products to be safe and our obligations to ensure this.

If you have any concerns about our products, you can contact us on ProductSafety@springernature.com

In case Publisher is established outside the EU, the EU authorized representative is:

Springer Nature Customer Service Center GmbH
Europaplatz 3
69115 Heidelberg, Germany

Batch number: 10755292

Printed by Printforce, the Netherlands